FIFTY SHADES OF

DUMB

Also by Leland Gregory:

FIFTY SHADES OF

DUMB

TRUE STORIES OF STRANGE AND SCREWY SEX

Leland Gregory

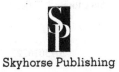

Skyhorse Publishing

Skyhorse Publishing books may be purchased in bulk at special discounts for sales promotion, corporate gifts, fund-raising, or educational purposes. Special editions can also be created to specifications. For details, contact the Special Sales Department, Skyhorse Publishing, 307 West 36th Street, 11th Floor, New York, NY 10018 or info@skyhorsepublishing.com.

Skyhorse® and Skyhorse Publishing® are registered trademarks of Skyhorse Publishing, Inc.®, a Delaware corporation.

Visit our website at www.skyhorsepublishing.com.

10 9 8 7 6 5 4 3

Library of Congress Cataloging-in-Publication Data

Gregory, Leland.

  Fifty shades of dumb : true stories of strange and screwy sex / Leland Gregory.
     pages cm
  ISBN 978-1-62636-016-7 (alk. paper)
  1. Sex--Humor. 2. Sex--Anecdotes. I. Title.
  PN6231.S54G69 2013
  818'.602--dc23

                            2013016227

Printed in the United States of America

This book is dedicated to all the long-suffering folks who have tolerated the whole *Fifty Shades of Grey* phenomenon, from the lonely husband listening to his wife giggle and moan in bed next to him, to the braces-wearing teen who thinks "dildo" is a character in *The Hobbit*. Whatever your take on *Fifty Shades of Grey*, that book pales in comparison to the real life events in *Fifty Shades of Dumb*. Truth is stranger than fiction . . . and less painful than friction. Enjoy.

"Sex is the most fun you can have without laughing." —Woody Allen

"Sex at age ninety is like trying to shoot pool with a rope." —George Burns

"Sex: the thing that takes up the least amount of time and causes the most amount of trouble." —John Barrymore

"I'll come and make love to you at five o'clock. If I'm late start without me." —Tallulah Bankhead

"I have no objection to anyone's sex life as long as they don't practice it in the street and frighten the horses." —Oscar Wilde

FIFTY SHADES OF

DUMB

Things That Go Bump in the Night

A middle-aged woman in England was awakened by a strange noise in her house and immediately called the police. The Bobbies arrived promptly and scoured the residence looking for the source of the sound. The woman's face went from "white with fear" to "red with embarrassment" when the police discovered an intruder of another sort caused the noise: the woman's sex-toy going off in her nightstand. A spokesperson for the police said the officers on call had a difficult time keeping a straight face when they apprehended the apparatus. I suppose the term "assault and battery" would apply here—for her next assault, she'll need new batteries.

Hey, Boo-Boo!

Charles Marshall was arrested in Cincinnati, Ohio, according to a June 15, 2012, report in the *Smoking Gun*, and charged with exposing himself and mimicking sex with a teddy bear. This was his fourth arrest in two years for the same offense. Talk about knocking the stuffing out of something.

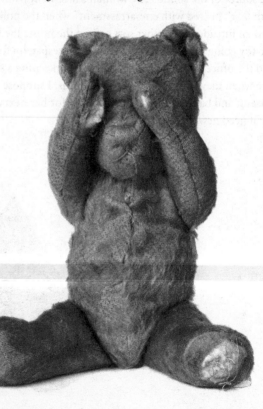

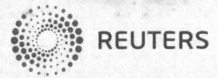

August 9, 2002

Does Sex Make Women Sprinters Faster??

Weenie Dog

On May 26, 2012, the *Moscow-Pullman Daily News* reported
that a thirty-six-year-old man was arrested in Harvard,
Idaho, and charged with indecent exposure. The man was taken
into custody after approaching a fenced dog, flashing
and wagging his penis, and trying to lure the dog over to
nuzzle (or muzzle) his genitals.

It Ain't Called a Jack-O-Lantern for Nothin'

In September 2002, a forty-five-year-old man in Warren, Michigan, was convicted of indecent exposure and sentenced to ninety days in jail. Police arrested Bill Patton after neighbors complained that he has naked in the backyard and was using a pumpkin to gratify himself sexually. When the man was approached by police, he blurted out, "What, is it midnight all ready?" (Sorry, I made that last part up.)

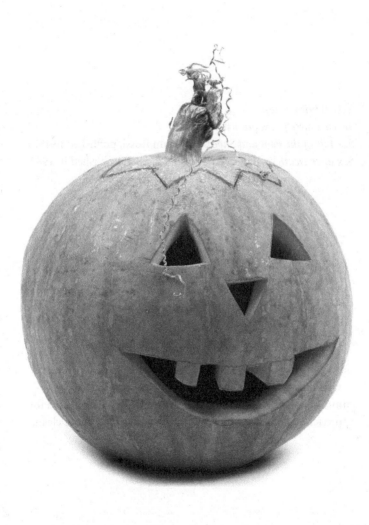

Actual book titles:
Teach Yourself Sex, published in 1951
Sex Life of the Foot and Shoe by William Rossi, published in 1977
Sex after Death by B. J. Ferrell and D. E. Frey, published in 1983

Spit Shine

According to a January 12, 2012, report on a television station in Glasgow, Scotland, Gary Paterson was sentenced to community service and psychotherapy after being convicted for approaching four boys and attempting to lick their shoes clean.

Every year, according to BizarreNews.com, eleven thousand Americans injure themselves while trying out bizarre sexual positions.

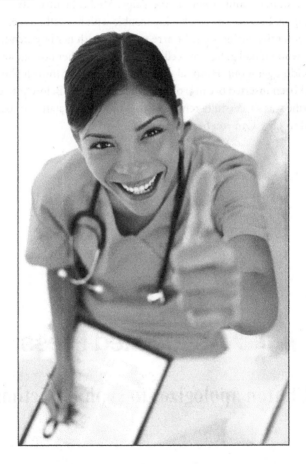

Loud and Clear

A Taiwanese woman went to the Taipei Medical University Hospital because she was having trouble with her cell phone. Apparently, during some bizarre sex game with her boyfriend, the woman had gotten the cell phone lodged in her bottom and couldn't get it out. Hospital staffers theorized that the cell phone had been inserted because of its vibrating feature. Before the cell phone was successfully removed, you know some staff member had to say, "Can you hear me now? Good!"

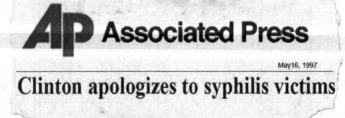

AP Associated Press

May16, 1997

Clinton apologizes to syphilis victims

Smokin' Hot

Passengers on a jam-packed train from Margate to Victoria, England, watched silently as John Henderson and Zoë D'Arcy engaged in oral sex and then moved on to intercourse. But, according to the August 7, 1992, article in the *Independent*, it wasn't until the couple lit up post-coital cigarettes that a number of people complained.

Abstinence advocate Pat Socia told a crowd of teenagers at a high school sex-education rally in Chicago in April 2000 that if they felt a sexual urge coming on, "Just eat a Snickers bar. You'll be fine!"

Hair Lip

On April 18, 2012, *Agence France-Presse* reported that fifty-year-old Tetsuya Ichikawa was arrested after approaching a twenty-five-year-old woman in a restaurant in Shizuoka, Japan, and licking her hair.

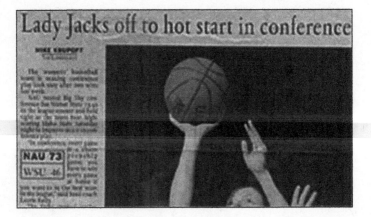

All in a Day's Work

According to a February 2002 article in the *Journal of Mundane Behavior* (no, I'm not making that up), a team of behavior specialists reported that boring sex has become a "global problem." Guest editor Kimberly Mahaffy, assistant professor of sociology at Millersville University of Pennsylvania, wrote that, "Mundane sex speaks to the 'truth' of our everyday experiences. The novelty and lust have been replaced by 'Can we do it before 10 p.m.?' 'Do I have to take my socks off?' 'Can I just lay here while you do the work?'"

According to a *BBC News* report on July 29, 2004, a Malawian, Africa, court convicted a Catholic priest and a nun of disorderly conduct after they were caught having sex at Lilongwe International Airport in a Toyota Corolla.

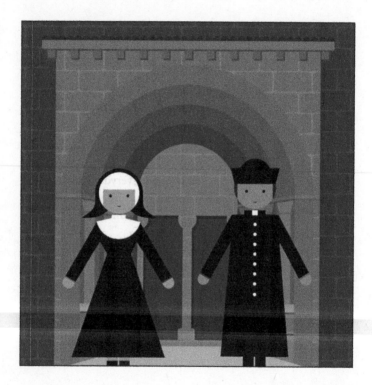

Mutton Mania

Charleston, West Virginia, police arrested Joey Armstrong on charges of trespassing, destruction of property, and cruelty to animals. According to a November 30, 2002, article in the *Charleston Daily Mail*, Armstrong apparently broke into a shed used to house animals for a live nativity scene at the Bartlett-Burdette-Cox Funeral Home and raped a sheep. Eventually he was sentenced to two years' probation and required to seek a mental health evaluation.

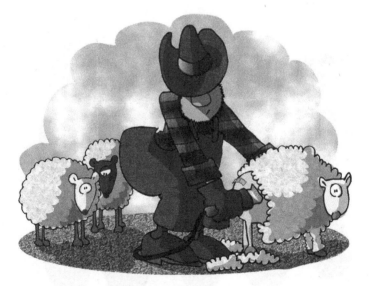

Out Standing in His Field

Robert Van Wagner of Port St. Lucie, Florida, was arrested after three girls (ages twelve and thirteen) reported to police that he tried to entice them to run around a field fully clothed. According to an April 29, 2012, article in the local newspaper, *TCPalm*, Wagner's only request was that they wear their socks but no shoes and allow him to watch. I wonder if the parents of the girls complained more about Wagner's actions, or how to get the grass stains out of their socks?

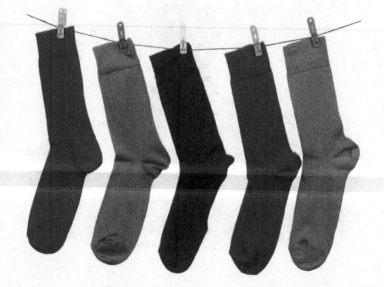

Once, Twice, Three Times a Lady...

In December 1997, a twenty-four-year-old woman in Beloit, Wisconsin, was charged with battery for allegedly hitting her husband with a plant stand, sending him to the hospital for six stitches. According to the police statement, the newlyweds frequently fought about sex. The night of the attack, the woman became enraged because her husband decided to call it quits after only four sexual encounters with her that day.

Car-Crossed Lovers

In July 1997, two "love birds" from Naples, Italy, were fooling around at a local lovers' lane in their subcompact car ("you put your foot in the glove box and I'll rest my elbow in the cup holder . . .") when they were accidentally hit from behind. The couple claimed they "lost control" during the collision and are suing for $100,000 to recover the expenses of their unplanned pregnancy. I guess the airbags weren't the only thing that deployed during the accident.

A Kodak Moment

On July 17, 2000, Elizabeth Whitaker and Aaron Caudill, both of Kentucky, stopped by a photo booth at Paramount's Kings Island Amusement Park near Cincinnati and couldn't help popping in and having their picture taken. Police reported that the man, "casually mentioned to his girlfriend that she could give him oral sex in this photo booth" and she did. According to an August 18, 2000, article in the *Cincinnati Enquirer*, things quickly developed from there—including a copy of the photographs prominently displayed on a monitor outside the booth. Once the blood came back to the man's brain, he realized what was going on and rushed outside to try to cover the monitor with his hands. The couple needed more than red-eye reduction after the incident, as they were arrested on charges of public indecency.

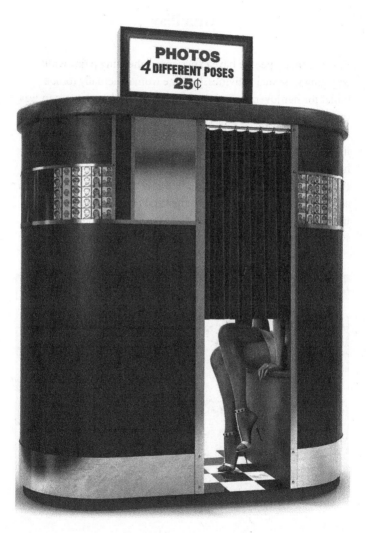

Gun Play

I'm sure many people have experienced shooting pains while engaging in sexual activities, but one woman actually took a bullet for her lover. A seventeen-year-old Pittsburgh woman was rushed to the hospital after her boyfriend went off half-cocked (actually his gun went off half-cocked). The couple was involved in some pretty bizarre "bedroom activities" when the .45-caliber handgun they were using as a prop fired and lodged a bullet in the woman's groin. The boyfriend was arrested and charged with aggravated assault, reckless endangerment, and corruption of a minor. It was believed the gun discharged accidentally, and I'm sure it was the only thing that discharged that evening.

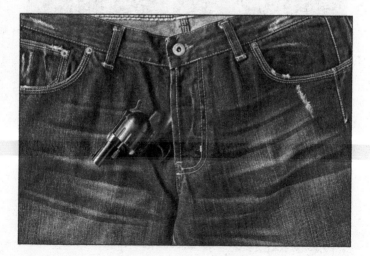

According to CODE §§61-8B-3 (enacted 1976), in West Virginia, "it is a felony for a person at least fourteen to engage in sexual intercourse, sexual intrusion, or sexual contact with a person under twelve."

Only the Lonely

Police in Stuttgart, Germany, responded to a call about a man and a woman having sex in a busy public shopping arcade and were sent to let the air out of the couple's passion. It was easier than they thought because the man's partner was full of hot air—in fact, she was a blow-up doll. According to a September 1, 2004, Reuters article, the intoxicated thirty-eight-year-old man was caught with his pants down and police had "considerable difficulty" separating him man from his latex companion. "It was real; he was caught in mid-action with the doll," said a press spokeswoman.

Return to Sender

Workers at a post office in Berlin, Germany, got quite a scare when one of the packages they were set to deliver started vibrating and making strange noises. Police accosted the man who had mailed the suspicious package, and he claimed it wasn't a bomb, but that the item did need to be blown up. The man admitted the package contained a life-size female sex doll with an electronic devise that vibrated and made "naughty" noises. The man said he was returning the doll to the manufacturer because it would spontaneously turn itself on at the most inopportune time—like at a post office. Postal authorities removed the batteries and sent the doll on her way. I hope they didn't send her third class—it would probably make her feel cheap.

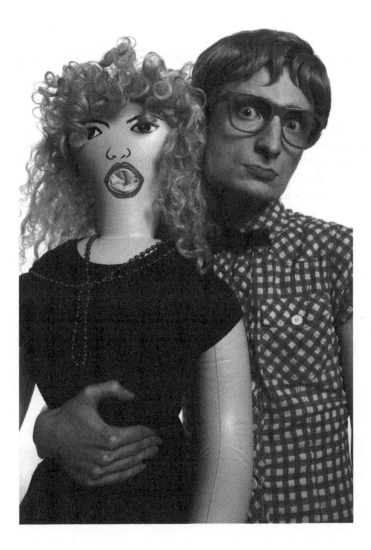

Winging It

Two "noisy" frequent fliers disturbed their fellow passengers on an overnight British Airways flight from Phoenix, Arizona, to London, England. The couple, an American man and a British woman, who were strangers before the flight, were taking full advantage of the fully reclining seats. After flight attendants asked the amorous couple to keep it down, they put everything in a fully upright and locked position. "We certainly would not encourage this sort of behavior," said a British Airways spokesman. "They obviously found our Club Class seats extremely comfortable."

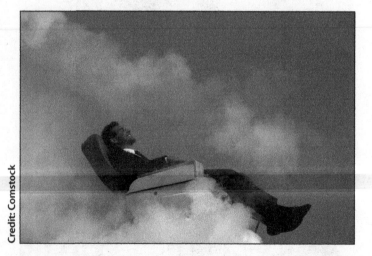

Credit: Comstock

Better than Nostradamus

A prostitute in Nagoya, Japan, had come up with a new trick for the oldest profession. The working girl, known only as Kaho (which, in and of itself, sounds like slang for a prostitute) claimed she could tell a man's future by having sex with him. According to a January 2000 article in the *Mainichi Daily News*, Kaho took credit for one of her customers winning at a racetrack and for encouraging a groom with cold feet to marry.

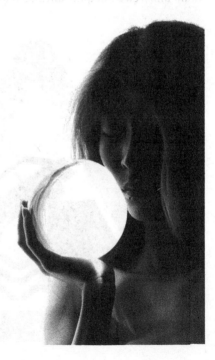

Going Down for a Second Time

A couple parked by the River Enns, near the city of Graz, Austria, went skinny-dipping—by accident. The unidentified man and woman had been making love for about fifteen minutes when they suddenly felt the car moving. According to a May 14, 2002, Ananova.com article, the handbrake wasn't set properly, and the car rolled down an embankment and into the icy river where it sank. The couple quickly uncoupled, escaped from the car, and swam unharmed but quite unclothed to the riverbank.

Boot Scooting

A burglar alarm summoned police one day to a western boot store in Bakersfield, California. When one of the officers looked in the large display window, he noticed there was more than just hand-tooled leather boots. According to an October 2004 article in the *Bakersfield Californian*, an officer tapped on the window to alert the two booty-bouncing burglars they were getting the boot. The couple took to their heels, but were quickly apprehended and charged with burglary, resisting an officer, assault on an officer, and indecent exposure. The two bootlicks admitted they had broken into the store to get out of the rain and then ducked into a "hidden" place to have sex. Seems that their mantra was not "If the shoe fits, wear it," but rather "If the boot fits, wear it out."

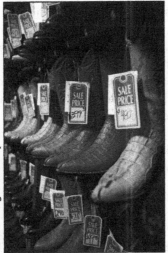

Credit: Kraig Scarbinsky

A German couple demanded $4,000 in damages from a tour operator because the maid at their hotel walked in on them twice while they were having sex, even though they had a "Do Not Disturb" sign hung on the door. I don't know who was more disturbed, the couple or the maid.

Survey Says!

A survey conducted in September 2005 by JWT Worldwide, a New York-based ad agency, and reported in a September 26, 2005, article from UPI, asked 2,126 English-speaking men and women in the United States, Britain, Canada, and the Netherlands a series of questions regarding sex. Unfortunately for Canadians, Canada ranks number one in terms of female sexual dissatisfaction. Of the 1,034 participating Canadians, 43 percent of the women said "sex is overrated" and 29 percent of the men agreed with the statement. In addition to this ego-deflating news is that while 81 percent of the Canadian women claim they have become more proactive in bed, 65 percent of the men and women in Canada argued that females have gotten "more demanding in bed."

The name of Texas A&M University researcher who conducted a study on teenage abstinence programs? Buzz Pruitt.

Man of the Year Award

Caller: "Can you tell me what happened to my girlfriend?"
911 Dispatcher: "I will try."
Caller: "Well, we were having sex. We really started going at it, and she started breathing hard and then passed out at the end. I thought she wasn't breathing so I started doing CPR on her. She came to. She is sleeping now and I think she is fine but I just wanted to know what happened to her?"
911 Dispatcher: "Sir, I think it was just *you*. If you want I can send a medic truck over to see if she is okay."
Caller: "Oh no, she is sleeping now. I think she should be all right in the morning."

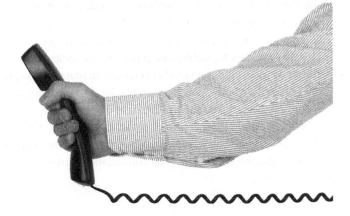

Damn Sand Gets into Everything

Imagine the surprise of dozens of beach goers out for a relaxing day at Mentor Headlands State Park Beach on Lake Erie near Cleveland, Ohio. They unfolded their blankets, got out their picnic baskets, and checked out the beautiful surroundings: the beach, the sparkling waters of the lake, the couple having sex. Apparently, Jim Santoro and Judith Reichel were bobbing up and down, but they weren't in the water. Several families complained to lifeguards and the couple were arrested and hauled into the courtroom of Painesville Judge Michael Cicconetti. The judge gave the couple a choice: They could either go to jail for twenty-two days for public indecency or they could make a public apology. As they had publicly engaged in oral sex, this gag order required them to publish ads in two local newspapers, with the wording, "I apologize for any activities that I engaged in that were offensive and disrespectful." I'm sure the ads about their June 13, 2002, tryst will be an interesting addition to the couple's scrapbook and will make for a great conversation starter.

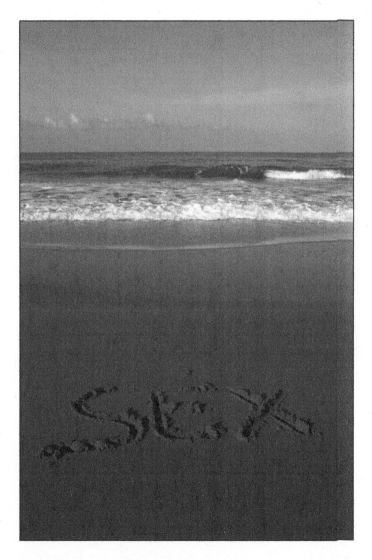

A Real Quickie

Usually when a policeman pulls a car over for speeding he's ready to hear some crazy excuses. But when a Montana Highway Patrol officer pulled over the speeding car of Robert Niel Johnson, of Illinois, the man didn't try to hide anything. "How come you don't have your pants on?" officer Darvin Mees asked Johnson. The officer then glanced over at the passenger, Shelby Kauffman, who was a little more discrete, Mees observed, for she "somewhat has her pants on." The woman, who couldn't keep her lips zipped either, told the officer that she and Johnson had just gotten engaged and started "getting frisky" in the car. According to CBSNews.com's "The Odd Truth, February 23, 2004," Mees asked the man to get out of the car and when he saw the driver stumble, he arrested him. After only fifteen minutes of deliberation, the jury in Johnson's drunk driving trial threw the charge out citing a lack of evidence. "Anybody caught with their pants down like that would be nervous," the jury's foreman said.

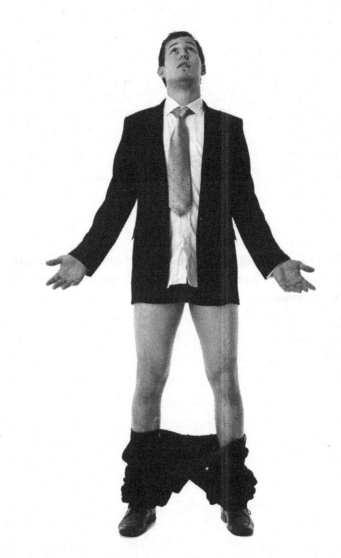

A fifty-two-year-old woman in the Italian town of Chieti divorced her ninety-four-year-old husband after only five months—because he demanded too much sex.

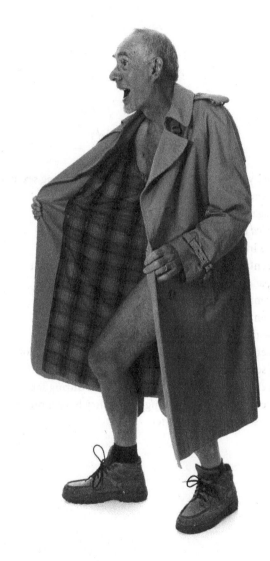

Rank and File

Just in case you want to know your chances of having sex at a certain location, and other specifics, the fine folks at *Brides* magazine (June 1998 issue), along with the book, *Just Married* by Barry Sinrod (yes, that's his real name) have some interesting stats:

- 60 percent of couples admit they don't have sex when staying at either partner's parents' house
- 70 percent claim they mess around while driving
- 17 percent of young married couples actually "did the deed" on their very first date
- 31 percent have admitted to the somewhat creepy act of having sex with a sleeping partner
- 64 percent say they don't have to be kissed during sex
- 67 percent reported, surprisingly, that they have more sex before marriage than after

That's Good Mood Food

A couple pleaded no contest to a charge of public indecency for engaging in sex in a booth at a Hardee's restaurant in New Philadelphia, Ohio. During the hearing, the prosecutor told the judge that although this was the couple's first lewdness charge, it was not the first time they had "done something like that." According to a June 30, 2003, article in the *Nation's Restaurant News*, the judge told the couple they should grow up and act their age: the man was seventy and the woman was sixty. The people at the Hardee's restaurant became suspicious when the woman kept yelling what they thought was, "Hardee's! Hardee's!" and then realized she was commenting on more than his Thickburger.

According to the May 2003 *City Pages of Minneapolis,* nurses took down the following comments from patients they saw in Room 111 for the treatment of sexually transmitted diseases:

"Burnin' when I urine."

"This guy I had sex with—his penis looked funny, kinda like a little pickle."

"Gots the gonga."

"Last time I had sex, I passed something that looked like cream of wheat before it's cooked."

"I got a bump on my little pearl."

"How am I supposed to do lap dances smelling like a dead fish?"

"Had sex with my daughter's fiancée and then douched with Lysol."

"Sex with over six hundred women, but it's not my fault."

"I used to have a trophy dick. Now I can't even look at it."

Auto-Erotic Asphyxiation

Jose Agustin Noh, an employee of the Perez Diaz funeral home, and Ana Maria Camara Suarez of Campeche, Mexico, died in 1999 from carbon monoxide poisoning after having sex in an automobile. To cool things down while things heated up, they left the engine running to keep the air conditioning on. After carpulating, they fell asleep and eventually succumbed to the carbon monoxide fumes. What makes this story particularly strange is that the car they had sex in and then died in was a hearse. I guess having sex in a hearse isn't too bizarre—it is referred to as a "bone wagon," anyway, right?

A Real Crush

Bryan Loudermilk of Okeechobee, Florida, died in a most peculiar fashion and police began an investigation. After questioning the deceased's wife, Stephanie Loudermilk, at length, detectives finally ruled Bryan's death as accidental. Apparently Bryan was a victim of a sexual fetish gone wrong. It was reported in an April 20, 2006, article in the *Broward Palm Beach New Times* that Bryan's body was found in a specially constructed pit, that a board had been placed over him, and that the rear wheel of the couple's red 1994 Honda Passport was parked on top of him. Police believe that Bryan received erotic thrills from being run over. I suppose when his wife told people she still had a crush on her husband, she meant something completely different.

What's Good for The Goose . . .

According to Minnesota Statute 609.36, 1963, adultery occurs when a married woman has sexual intercourse with a man other than her husband, whether the man is married or not. Both parties are guilty of a misdemeanor. A prosecution for adultery requires a complaint by a spouse of one of the offenders, unless those spouses are insane. It is a defense to adultery that the man did not know the marital status of the woman. There is no prohibition against sex between a married man and an unmarried woman.

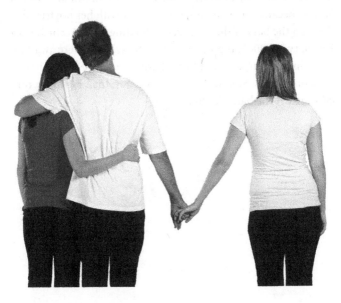

Jail House Rocks!

We've all seen movies where prisoners secretly exchange things through the bars of their cells. But one couple in Britain's Swansea Crown Court building passed something through the bars that you would only see in a *different* kind of prison movie. An investigation was launched when an inmate, Donna Stokes, became pregnant after having sex with her boyfriend through the bars of their respective holding cells. According to a February 18, 2000, report from BBC News, both were awaiting a hearing on burglary and theft charges and were in adjoining temporary cells. Sounds like a lot more fun than rattling a tin cup against the bars, doesn't it?

An old statute in Kentucky reads: "A man shall not marry the grandmother of his wife."

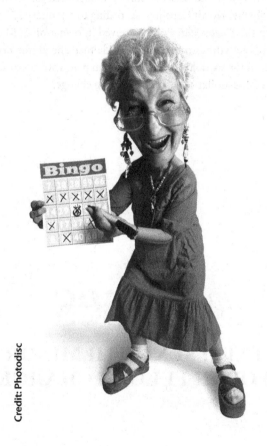

Every Penny Counts

Twenty-five-year-old Misty Kullman was arrested for prostitution in Shelby, North Carolina, according to a January 25, 2012, article in the *Shelby Star*. Police received information of Ms. Kullman's activities from a man who claimed she performed oral sex on him for six dollars, which the man paid with a two-dollar bill, three one-dollar bills, and the rest in change.

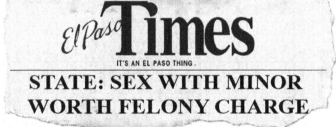

STATE: SEX WITH MINOR WORTH FELONY CHARGE

As You Sow So Shall You Reap

ABC News reported on October 20, 2000, about a couple from Brnicko, Czechoslovakia, who were enjoying a roll in the hay when it suddenly became a roll and a "Hey!" While sowing some wild oats in a field, they heard a noise that made their brows furrow. It was the terrifying sound of a farmer on a tractor taking a short cut through his field. The farmer did more than just take a short cut; he also cut the couple up fairly well, causing severe injuries to the woman's chest and the man's buttocks. The nearly-cropped couple tried to keep the accident a secret, as they were embarrassed and unmarried, but doctors and insurers tracked down the origin of their injuries. That's what happens in a relationship when there's an attractee and a-tractor.

Coke and a Smile

US Air Force Capt. Jacqueline Chester tested positive for cocaine and was brought before a court martial tribunal in Dover, Delaware. Coming to her defense was Charles Gittins, her ex-husband, who testified that during their marriage, to prolong his erection and increase his pleasure, he would occasionally rub cocaine on his genitals. According to a January 19, 2004, article in the *Air Force Times*, Gittins proposed that since Jacqueline never used drugs, she must have absorbed the drug through her vaginal walls.

According to a Maryland Code (Article 27, §3, enacted in 1749) that is still on the books, adultery is considered a misdemeanor, but punishable only by a $10 fine.

Sleeping Beauty

According to the Dubuque, Iowa, *Telegraph-Herald*, Jeannie M. Patrinos was sentenced in February 2003 to five years' probation for sexual assault. Patrinos, who was estranged from her husband, broke into his home, climbed into bed with him, and was caught "having sex" with him against his will by the man's girlfriend, who was sleeping beside him in the same bed at the time.

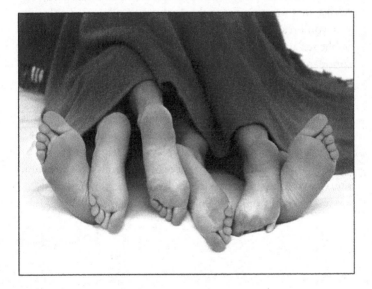

Come and Go

The criminal complaint against Joseph Sivertsen of Spenard, Alaska, that was reported in the *Anchorage Daily* is something you won't read every day: "Spontaneous interruption of a public sex act to engage in an aggravated assault should be considered as a strong indication of a seriously unaddressed anger management problem." In June 2002, pedestrian Jerome King spotted Joseph and his girlfriend having sex in an alley way and asked the pair, "Are you having fun?" Joseph, who up to that point probably was having fun, became infuriated at the private remark about his public display of affection. Witnesses reported that Joseph grabbed a piece of pipe from a construction site, chased King into a parking lot, and struck him repeatedly. So Joseph went from laying pipe to swinging pipe.

Love Thyself

At an academic conference on sexuality in Madison, Wisconsin, Robert Bahr, the founder of a newsletter on masturbation, explained that some of his readers had adopted a "solo" sexual orientation (which differs from hetero, homo, or bi-sexual orientation). In a September 1999 article in *Canada's National Post*, Bahr commented that some of his readers, not unlike the Greek myth of Narcissus, "have fallen in love with their own reflections." Some engage in "marathons of masturbation, honeymoons in which they lock themselves away in their own homes, parading naked from mirror to mirror."

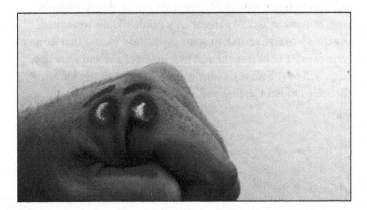

O, I Understand

The German chemical and pharmaceutical company Bayer
conducted a survey of men in Finland in September 2005 and
gathered some interesting facts on orgasms. According to the
survey's findings, most men think it's "of utmost importance"
that their partner achieve orgasm during sex. Sounds like those
Finnish men are compassionate lovers, right? Well, the survey
went on to reveal that 25 percent didn't think female orgasms
were important and 10 percent either didn't know what these
orgasms looked like and, in some cases, didn't know that women
were capable of having them. The women of Finland were not
surprised by the survey's conclusions. They've always known
their men to Finnish first and ask questions later.

Balls in Your Court

A January 13, 2012, article in the *Minneapolis News City Pages* explained that authorities had finally let the air out of the weird fetish of Christopher Bjerkness of Duluth, Minnesota. He was sentenced to twenty-three months in prison, but this was converted to four years of supervised probation. His problem? Bjerkness has been arrested several times for breaking into various establishments and slashing rubber exercise balls. In 2005, Bjerkness damaged forty exercise balls in the University of Minnesota Duluth's sports complex, and in 2006, he hacked up seventy balls at the Polinsky Medical Rehabilitation Center. Three years later, Bjerkness broke into SMDC-Duluth Clinic West building and slashed the rubber balls there. Bjerkness admitted he had an unstoppable and unexplainable sexual urge to destroy the balls.

Now *That* Sucks

The Item from Sumter, South Carolina, reported on May 13, 1998 about a classic case of "It seemed like a good idea at the time." A fifty-one-year-old Long Branch, New Jersey, man screamed "Eureka!" after he stuck his penis in his vacuum cleaner. The vacuum had more than cleaned his high-traffic areas; it had also chopped off a half inch of the drunken man's penis. When officers first arrived on the scene, the man tried to convince them he had been stabbed in the crotch as he slept. But Long Branch public safety director Louis Napoletano soon realized the man had tried to put his own "attachment" in the vacuum. "But what he didn't realize," Napoletano said, "is that there's a blade in the vacuum cleaner right under where the hose attaches that pushes the dust into the collection bag." The rest of the man's "hose" was found in the collection bag, but doctors were unable to reattach it.
I guess the Dyson Ball Vacuum doesn't mean what some people think it does.

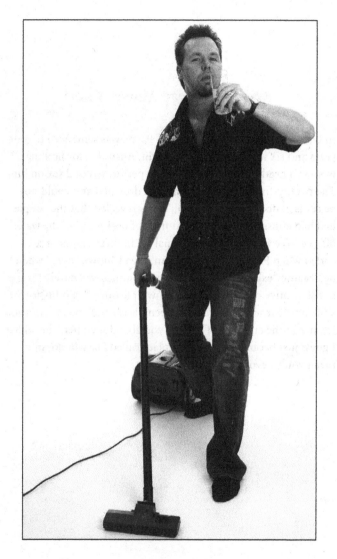

Keep Your Head Above Water!

In October 1997, Christopher Sean Payne was sentenced to four years and six months in jail in Darwin, Australia, for holding a woman's head under water while she performed oral sex on him. The twenty-five-year-old woman had drowned and could not be resuscitated. During the trial, it was revealed that the couple had had consensual sex "in a number of positions" in the water off Pee Wee Camp Beach. The final act in their drama of sex ended when Payne held the woman's head "down there" when he became "excited." "Your criminal conduct was purely for the selfish motive of continuing your own pleasure," said Justice Sir William Kearney. "She had just been pleasuring you . . . And you left her in the embrace of the sea; you abandoned her," he added. I guess just because you live in a place called Darwin doesn't mean you've evolved.

According to the *Calgary Sun*, Gerald Allan Naud, a former pro boxer in Edmonton, Canada, pleaded guilty to sexual assault in 2004 after harassing women to kick him in the balls.

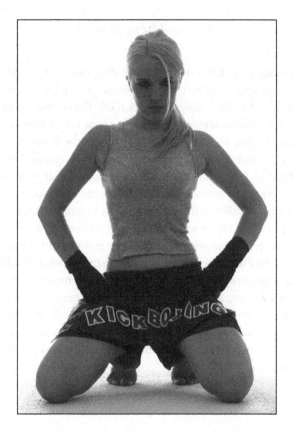

I'll Be There in a Jif

While engaging in BDSM games, a Bremerton, Washington, man suggested to his wife that they smear peanut butter over his genitals and let their Irish Setter lick it off. The couple did just that, and all three seemed to have a fine time for a while—until the dog became more excited than anyone at the prospect of eating as much peanut butter as he wanted. The dog decided to dig right in, fangs and all, and started biting and tearing at the man's penis and testicles. Needless to say, the man didn't enjoy feeling his testicles go from extra crunchy to gone. His wife added insult to injury when she sprayed perfume at the dog, trying to get him to release his grip. The perfume only intensified her husband's pain when it hit his mangled penis. Finally, the dog ran away with a portion of penis in his mouth, and the man passed out. The wife packed the dismembered part of his member in a Styrofoam cooler, took him to the hospital, and doctors successfully rewired his wang. One thing is certain: I'll bet the man gets an odd feeling every time he sees his dog chewing on a bone.

I'm Lovin' It!

According to a January 16, 2012, article in the *Burbank Leader*, a Ms. Khadijah Baseer was arrested in Los Angeles on suspicion of prostitution. Several men came forward and accused Baseer of opening their car doors while they were in the drive-thru lane at a McDonald's and offering to perform oral sex on them in exchange for Chicken McNuggets.

"Call for Submissions: Sex Worker Anthology." Soft Skull Press released this ad in 2005, looking for contributors for an anthology of stories by sex trade workers. The ad solicited strippers, whores, hustlers, escorts, film, or print models.

Letting the Air out of a Relationship

A Brazilian man was so incensed when his parents demanded he divorce his wife that he went on a killing spree. While arguing with her son over his choice of brides, the seventy-one-year-old mother grabbed a pair of scissors and lunged at the man's "wife." He wrestled the scissors from her hands and murdered both her and his father on the spot. Turns out the wife was a doll—literally. Police said the man "thought the doll was a human being, called her his bride and talked to her," a family acquaintance said. The man was taken to jail, and his wife was utterly deflated.

Fox News reported on August 30, 2001, that a *Journal of Sex Research* report by two Georgia State University professors concluded that people who want sex but are not getting any are grumpier than those who are having sex or even those who don't desire it. From the fine folks who brought you Duh!

That Takes the Cake

A couple in Craiova, Romania, as reported in *Ananova* on April 19, 2002, went to the hospital as a result of what could only be described as "Laurel and Hardy have sex." The comic chain of events occurred while the man was cooking pancakes and his girlfriend decided it would be fun to perform oral sex on him. As he focused less and less on the pancakes, the man accidentally spilled hot oil on the woman's back. She instinctively bit down hard, and when she raised her head up, she bonked her head on the bottom of the frying pan he was holding. The man was treated for severe bites while his girlfriend was treated for burns on her back and a laceration on her scalp. Doctors listed the cause of the couple's wounds as head injury.

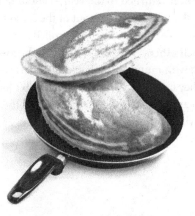

In November 2000, *Ananova* reported the same series of events happening to a couple in Bucharest while the man was cooking french fries.

Lost and Found

In Dennis, Massachusetts, a police officer assisted a honey-mooning couple who had lost their way by giving them directions. The female driver thanked the officer, who then got back into her patrol car and drove off. Not much of a story so far, right? Well, it gets better. According to a police spokesman, who was quoted in a May 20, 2003, article in the *Boston Herald*, "When the officer returned to the vehicle about ten minutes later, she saw the female hanging out of the car and the male jump on the female." Then the couple rolled onto the highway "punching each other." The officer arrested the lovebirds and charged them with mutual assault and disorderly conduct. Apparently they couldn't stay mad at each other long though. "They had an amorous reunion in the lobby of the police station, to the point where officers had to separate them again but in a different way."

Super Sex

According to Cosmopolitan.com, a woman explained how she and her boyfriend were really into a particular lubricant. "One night we were both a little tipsy," she said, "and I told him I left it on my desk. He goes to put it on me and very quickly we both realized he had just put SuperGlue on my vagina, which must have been sitting next to it. He was able to pull his fingers off, but a part of my pretty newly waxed labia was already stuck together and couldn't be pulled apart. It was so bad and painful, I had to go the college hospital and even called my mom to come and console me!"

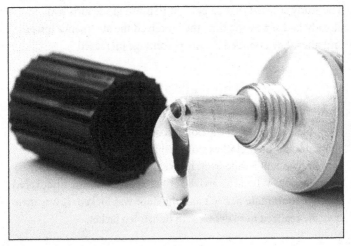

A study conducted by Advocates for Youth, published in 2000, gave a bad grade to the abstinence-only sex education programs in Texas schools (spearheaded by then Governor George Bush). The study showed that 23 percent of ninth grade girls had already had sex by the time they received the abstinence lessons, and after they attended . . . the percentage increased.

The Walk of Shame

A couple having sex in the Bon Accord Terrace Gardens in Scotland had their clothes stolen while they were doing it. The woman was half a mile from home and had only a newspaper to cover herself. When she arrived at her apartment, she discovered that her roommate had left and the door was locked. It was then that she realized her keys were in her stolen jacket.

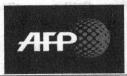

November 29, 2004

**Pig Not Degraded by Televised
Sexual Experience,
British Watchdog Rules**

A Graham of Goodness

Presbyterian minister Rev. Sylvester Graham developed the graham cracker in Bound Brook, New Jersey, in 1822, but it wasn't to complete the recipe for s'mores. In fact, it was created so that people wouldn't want s'more of anything—especially sex. Graham believed his cracker, along with bland foods and a strict vegetarian diet, could cure not only alcoholism but more importantly, sexual urges (which he believed to be the source of many maladies). Graham's belief that eating pure foods created a purity of mind, spirit, and body influenced several people, including Dr. John Harvey Kellogg, the inventor of the corn flakes breakfast cereal.

A Rose by Any Other Name

The Benton County Sheriff's Office received a tip about a man who had child pornography on his computer and they, along with the Arkansas State Police, investigated, secured a warrant, and searched the man's computer. According to a March 6, 2012, article in the *Arkansas Democrat-Gazette*, the arrested man's name was . . . wait for it . . . Dinky J. Head.

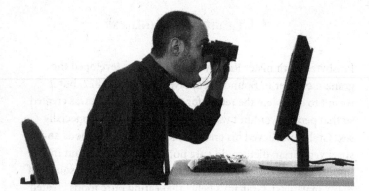

Out of Tune

According to a December 29, 2011, article in Tacoma Washington's newspaper the *News Tribune*, thirty-seven-year-old music teacher Kevin Gausepohl tried to convince one of his seventeen-year-old students that she would sing better if she tried it naked. The student complied with a few of Gausepohl's requests, but eventually turned him in. During his conviction for communicating with a minor for immoral purposes, Gausepohl tried to defend his actions by stating that he was experimenting at the "human participant level" in an effort to tune into the effects of vocal range on sexual arousal.

Spit in the Face of Justice

Forty-one-year-old Charles Hersel was accused of child molestation after he admitted to paying high school students to yell profanities at him, spit in his face, and urinate and defecate on him. However, during his trial, jurors decided that Hersel's bizarre requests must have stemmed from something other than "sexual gratification" purposes. According to a February 21, 2012, report on Los Angeles's KTLA-TV, technically, the jury deduced, Hersel wasn't in violation of California's child molestation statutes and he was acquitted.

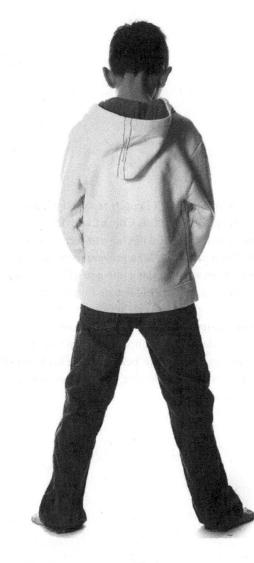

Dog Days

According to an April 6, 2012, Reuters report, the Kansas Supreme Court ruled that Joshua Coman, convicted of having carnal relations with a dog, did not have to register as a sex offender. While on probation for a previous bestiality charge, Coman was arrested after breaking into a neighbor's garage and having sex with her four-year-old female Rottweiler. However, the Court gave Coman a long leash, because only felons have to register as sex offenders, and Coman was convicted of a misdemeanor. Coman also wasn't convicted of burglary, according to the judge, because, as he broke into the garage only to have sex with the dog, there was no intent to commit a felony or theft.

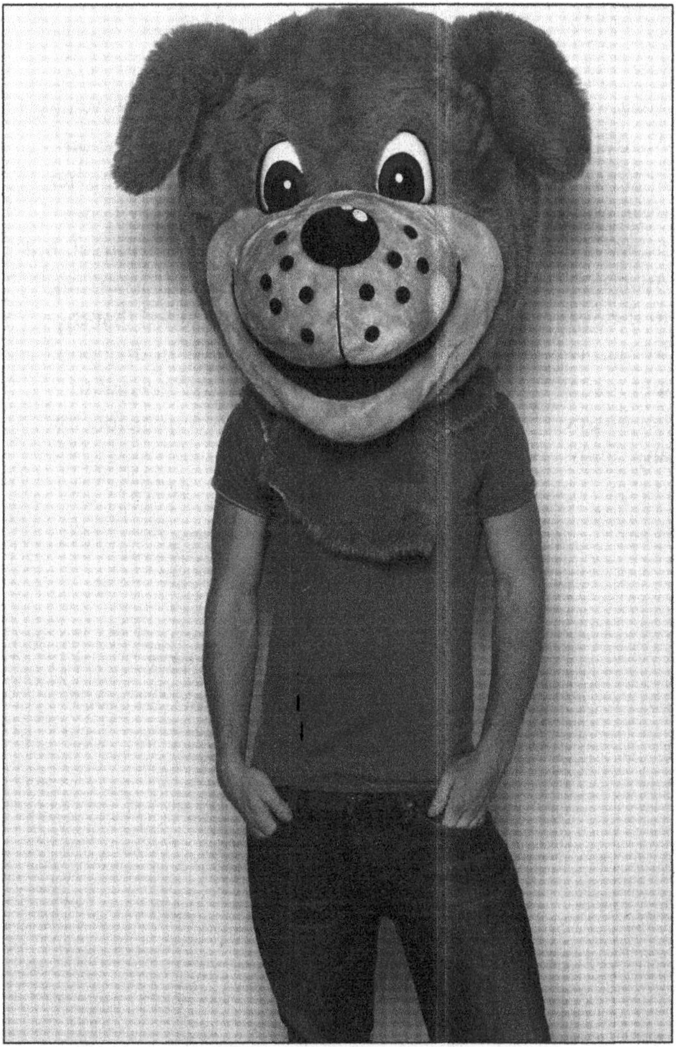

Nice Work If You Can Get It

A woman who was traveling on business in New South Wales, Australia, was injured while have wild sex in her hotel room in November 2007. A wall sconce had come loose during her tryst, and she was hurt. When she applied for worker's compensation, she was denied by the workplace safety tribunal. But Australia's Federal Court overturned the decision, according to the *Sydney Morning Herald*. The court concluded that the woman was in the city on business, and her stay in the hotel and sexual activity were all "ordinary incidents" related to her business, and therefore her company was responsible for any injuries.

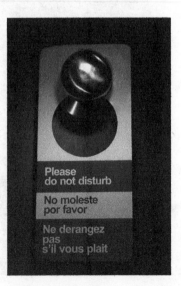

See What Develops

While standing at a urinal in a Trinity, Texas, bathroom, a fifty-seven-year-old man noticed that someone was taking a picture of him by holding a cellphone under the stall that was adjacent to the urinals. Chris Windham was arrested and charged with improperly photographing the man, but claimed, in his defense, that it was an accident. According to a March 20, 2012, article in the *Houston Press*, Windham explained that he typically balances himself on one hand while whipping himself with the other. He stated that during the alleged incident, he just happened to be holding his cellphone in the hand with which he braces himself.

Puppy Love

The *Local*, a German newspaper, reported on February 3, 2012, that Madeleine Martin, the animal protection official for the Hessian state government, claimed that her country desperately needed "stronger" anti-bestiality laws. Why? Because, she said, of the proliferation of "animal brothels" in Germany. And she's not talking about animal-on-animal sex.

Martin demanded new anti-bestiality laws because in order to convict under the existing laws, it must be proven not just that the animal was sexually violated by a person, but that violation caused the animal physical harm.

Old Yeller

An unnamed sixteen-year-old boy from Harris County, Texas, was charged with aggravated assault after shooting his father, Jacob Hughes, because he was convinced his father was hurting his mother. According to a February 14, 2005, article in the *Houston Chronicle*, the couple's eleven-year-old son was awakened around 3 a.m. to the sound of his mother screaming and moaning in his parents' bedroom. He woke up his older brother, who then ran into his parents' room, demanded his father to stop hurting his mom, and then shot his father in the arm. The sheriff's deputies arrived on the scene and were told that mom and dad hadn't been fighting . . . they had simply been engaging in consensual, albeit loud, sex.

Norway? Yes, Way!

There's a first time for everything, and in Norway for the first
time, a woman was convicted of raping a man. The unnamed
twenty-three-year-old woman was convicted of performing oral
sex on a sleeping thirty-one-year-old man. The Bergen court
sentenced the succubus to nine months in prison and fined her
the equivalent of $6,390. Although the woman confessed
to the immoral oral, she claimed that the man was not only
willing but was also smiling on that January 4, 2004, night.
The man, however, disagreed and asserted that the incident
frightened him to such a degree that it caused him psychological
problems and mental anguish.

The Key to a Lasting Relationship

While playing bondage games in a tent at a local campsite in Hampshire, England, a police officer handcuffed his girlfriend but lost the key. The man was forced to leave his girlfriend cuffed while he huffed off to a nearby police station to beg a spare. Police Federation chairman Alan Gordon was able to put a positive spin on the situation, stating in a meeting: "It is encouraging that our specials take their training seriously, not least the officer who had to borrow a handcuff key while off-duty."

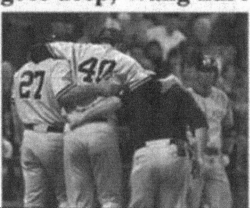

A-Rod goes deep, Wang hurt

By CHRIS DUNCAN
AP Sports Writer

HOUSTON — Chien-Ming Wang pitched five scoreless innings before spraining his right foot running the bases, and Alex Rodriguez hit a three-run homer in the New York Yankees' 13-0 win over the Houston for time on Sunday.

Wang (8-2) pulled up as he rounded third on Derek Jeter's two-run single during the Yankees' eight-run sixth inning. He hopped the rest of the way home and pointed to his right foot after scoring. A trainer rushed from the dugout to check on him and Wang was helped off the field.

Getting a rare chance to hit against an NL team, Wang had reached base on a bunt that turned into a...

Law of the Land

The fine folks on the city council wanted to reign in the burgeoning sex market in the progressive town of Clarksville, Tennessee, so they passed a city ordinance that prohibited operators of any "adult bookstore" from engaging in sex on the premises of the store. (There was only one adult bookstore in Clarksville in June 1995.) But in the council's haste, they left out the phrase "on the premises," thus making it illegal for the owner and his employees from having sex anywhere.

Slip and Slide

During his bachelor party, Justin Scheidt consented to get on the stage, lay on his back with his legs around the dance pole, and allowed several strippers to slide down the pole onto his crotch. After the incident, Scheidt complained that he had suffered "serious and permanent injuries" to his nether regions and filed a lawsuit against the Showgirl III strip club in Fort Wayne, Indiana. According to a May 16, 2003, article in the *Fort Wayne Journal Gazette*, the day following the groin grinding, Scheidt went ahead with his wedding, but claimed, because of his injuries, that he was unable to consummate the marriage.

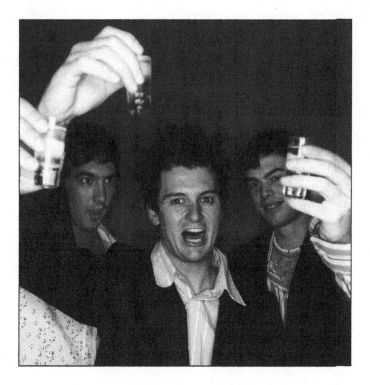

Stop, Shot, and Roll

Jimmy Watkins was found guilty of murdering his wife after
he discovered she was seeing another man. During his trial,
Watkins claimed he was overcome with anger and acted out of
"sudden passion" in shooting his cheating wife, Nancy, and her
paramour, Keith Fontenot. According to an October 22, 1999,
Associated Press article, the jury accepted Wakins's defense and
sentenced him to four months in jail even though after shooting
his wife once in the head, he shot Fontenot three times until
his gun jammed. Thinking he was out of bullets, he got into his
truck and drove away until he realized that there were more bullets in the magazine. He turned around, went back to the house,
and shot his wife again while she was calling 911.

Never Tire of Love

In January 2000, Frederick Alex Hunchak pled guilty in Wynyard, Saskatchewan, to purposely puncturing the tires of three cars. Hunchak admitted that he knew women drove all the cars and his plot was to "rescue" them by volunteering to change their damaged tires in the hope of finding true love.

A woman from New York City was convicted of trying to use her estranged husband's health insurance to get her current lover a penile implant.

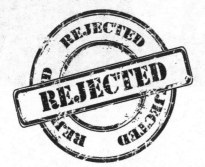

When Pigs Fly

Brian Pellow succeeded in a Supreme Court claim for negligence against Dawone Pty Ltd., proprietors of Jake's Piggery in New South Wales, Australia. According to a November 6, 1997 article from *Agence France-Presse*, the judge awarded the equivalent of $432,000 to the fifty-four-year-old man who claimed he lost his sex drive after being attacked by a pig. The judge was quoted as saying, "He . . . also has difficulty sleeping, driving his manual car, and has lost his libido."

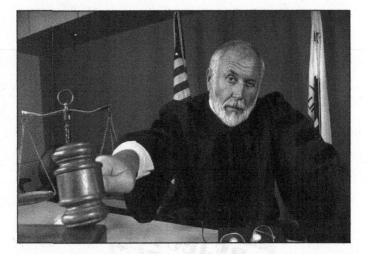

The Bride was a Real Dog

A groom-to-be loaned out his camera to a friend to videotape
his upcoming wedding, but inadvertently forgot to erase
the tape first. Wedding guests gathered around to watch a
replay of the ceremony but were dog-faced when they saw
the fifty-nine-year-old groom having sex with his neighbor's
bull terrier named Ronnie. According to a March 15, 1994,
Reuters article, the British man was found guilty of bestiality
even though he claimed that the ten-minute video was actually
an attempt at trick photography and only featured simulated sex acts.

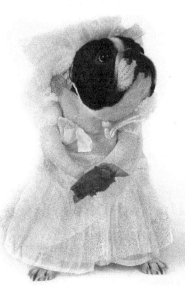

You're Only as Old as You Feel

A ninety-year-old man called the Charlotte, North Carolina, emergency center to complain of consumer fraud. He told the shocked dispatcher that he had recently hired a prostitute and she left him, well, dissatisfied. He wanted to file a formal complaint, have the prostitute arrested, and get his money back. When the dispatcher explained to the man that solicitation of prostitution was a crime, he quickly hung up. Makes you wonder if he got an AARP discount.

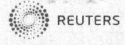 REUTERS

December 2, 2001

Sex Up and Down after September 11

Knife and Spoon

According to *Christopher Offord v. the State of Florida*, Offord refused the request of his wife, Dana Noser, to come back to bed after they had engaged in sex. According to the police interrogation, Offord "retrieved a knife and duct tape from the kitchen and went back to the bedroom. Offord sat down on the bed next to Noser and she continued to insist that he lie down. Offord took a piece of duct tape, put it over Noser's mouth, and began to hit her with his fist. The duct tape did not cover her entire mouth so he grabbed a pillow to muffle her. He repeatedly told Noser to 'shut up.' He grabbed the knife and began to stab Noser in the face and chest. Offord then saw the hammer beside the bed and started hitting her face with it. Offord stated that he hit Noser about fifty times with the hammer and that he believed he eventually broke her neck." Circuit Judge Dedee Costello sentenced the hammer-wielding Offord to death, saying, "The defendant struck his wife approximately seventy individual blows after spending a happy interlude with her," the judge said. "Her desire to cuddle after sex does not justify the extremely violent, brutal response of the defendant." His death sentence was eventually reduced to life in prison without possibility of parole. If this guy hates spooning now, just wait until he goes to prison.

Don't Leave the Light On!

How did a father in Georgia discover that his underage daughter was having an affair with a twenty-eight-year-old police officer? The cop left his patrol car parked in their driveway, that's how. The father arrived home early from work one evening and found the policeman in his teenaged daughter's bed in what looked like a strip search. The now ex-officer admitted to the illegal relationship, saying that he met the young girl while volunteering at her high school as a coach.

"Girlie Mags must Stay Abreast of the Net" – *London Observer* headline, September 10, 2005

Let's Make A Deal

A Belfry, Kentucky, man named Wood Keesee filed a lawsuit against a forty-nine-year-old woman, demanding $1,500 or fifteen sessions of sex. Keesee, a former Pike County school board member, claims he had a "sex for money deal" with Victoria Howell, a Floyd Circuit Court deputy clerk, at $100 per session. Keesee claims he paid the woman $1,800, but they only had sex three times. "She owes me 15 sessions or $1,500," he wrote in his complaint. Howell's attorney, Clyde Johnson, said: "(My client) specifically and vehemently denies each and every statement and allegation of the complaint." According to a May 14, 1997, article in the *Daily News*, Johnson also stated that his client and Keesee were romantically involved, but when she broke off the relationship, "he didn't like that and now he's trying to harass her and to extort money from her." Keesee was previously charged with impersonating his cousin, Pike County Sheriff Charles "Fuzzy" Keesee.

The Law's the Law

According to Section 288a.f.1 of the California Penal Code, the penalty for oral sex in California is up to eight years in jail, whether you are married or not, provided that one of the two people involved is asleep. Also eight years for using a dildo.

Deadbeat Groom

Rarely would someone need permission from the president to get married, but things are a little different in France. Twenty-two-year-old Karen Jumeaux relied on an obscure French law that allowed her to marry her fiancé Anthony Maillot although he'd been dead for nearly two years. President Nicolas Sarkozy granted Jumeaux permission for a posthumous wedding because she could prove they were already planning to marry. According to a June 24, 2011, article in the *Daily Mail Reporter*, they met in 2007 and had a baby boy in 2009, shortly before Maillot's death in a car accident at the age of twenty.

In February 2011, another Frenchwoman, thirty-five-year-old Christelle Demichel, married her boyfriend, a former policeman, who had been killed by a drunk driver in September 2002.

Taking It on the Chin

According to the book, *Sexuality in America: Understanding our Sexual Values and Behavior* by Patricia Koch, there is a man named Michael Brown who refers to himself as a "piesexual." He becomes sexuality aroused with, you guessed it, pies. Brown is so into getting off on his just deserts that he even produces pie videos and hosts "bring your own pie" parties where people strip naked and throw pies at each other.

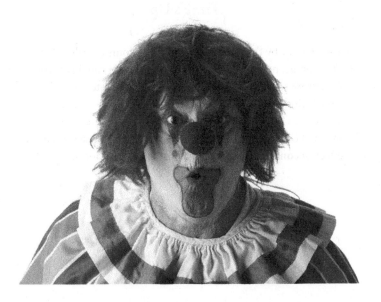

Time's Up

A 1998 survey by the makers of Durex condoms revealed that:
- On average, married couples have intercourse roughly forty fewer times per year than couples who cohabitate.
- Cohabiting couples also dedicate more time to lovemaking: averaging twenty-five minutes versus sixteen minutes for married couples. Of course, in my opinion, the desensitizing effect of condoms might count for the extra minutes.

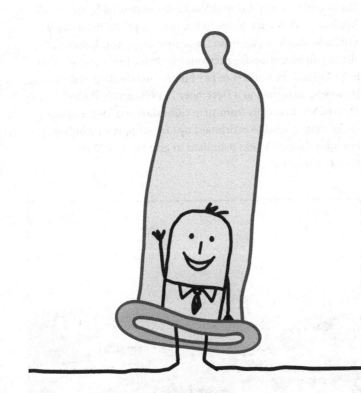

A Pig in a Poke

Thirty-eight-year-old Darrel Voeks was sentenced by an Appleton, Wisconsin, judge to ten years in prison for stealing $100,000 worth of pigs from his farmer-employer. Voeks, already on probation for previous pig thefts, told the court that he purloined the porkers to pay bills for his children and ex-wife. However, according to a December 7, 1996, article in the *Deseret News*, receipts from strip clubs showed that the majority of the money went to exorbitant tips for strippers, including one who claimed Voeks promised to give her $3,000 for breast implants.

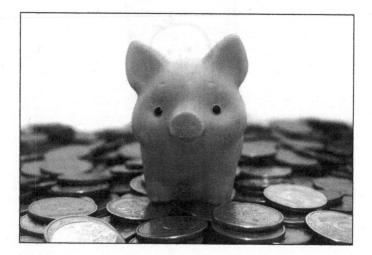

Taken for a Ride

According to an October 20, 1994, *Associated Press* article, the district court in Stockholm, Sweden, convicted a thirty-four-year-old taxi driver of overcharging an unnamed forty-nine-year-old woman after he took her for, euphemistically speaking, twenty-five rides. The man presented a written bill to the court laying out that the woman owed him the equivalent of $8,300 dollars for "sexual services." The bill also included expenses for trips, hotel rooms, telephone calls, and sales tax. The unnamed man was not charged with prostitution, as it is legal, but was convicted of overcharging the woman and sentenced to three years in prison.

It's What's for Dinner

It might not have been on the menu, but what one Orlando couple ordered certainly hit the spot. The manager of Paddy Murphy's restaurant called police after he "was notified by several patrons that a couple was having sex on a table in view of minor children," according to an Orlando Police Department report. According to an October 17, 2012, in the *Smoking Gun*, manager Tom Murphy approached the couple and demanded they stop their culinary copulation, to which the man, Jeremie Calo, responded, "She can't get up at this time." Calo tried to run out without paying his tab, but was restrained by restaurant employees until police arrived. The dining duo weren't prosecuted for their naughty table manners because, "the parents of the young children that observed Calo and Barganier having sex declined to write statements regarding their observations," investigating police reported. Now that's what I call "Dinner and a Show."

More and Mower

Delbert Buttrey was wanted in connection with kidnapping a transient couple from Indiana in July 1997. Police in Lexington, Kentucky, were on the look-out for Buttrey who, along with Buttrey's unnamed girlfriend, took the couple to an isolated location and forced them to perform oral sex on him while Buttrey's girlfriend took pictures. According to police, following the forced fellatio, Buttrey took the couple back to his home and made the man mow his lawn.

A Unique Butter Churn

Things were pretty quiet at 3 a.m. at the Sainsbury supermarket in Kensington, England, when Michael Pallant and his girlfriend, Danielle Minns, entered the store. The few shoppers there at the time smiled to themselves when they saw Minns in one of the shopping carts and Pallant pushing her down the aisle. When a security guard heard Minns scream, he ran to the back of the store, where he found the couple having sex in the dairy case, on top of the "margarine tubs, yoghurt, clotted cream and trifles," as he told the *New Straits Times*. When the security guard, who was more than just lactose intolerant, asked what the couple was doing, Pallant replied, "chilling out." They were fined the equivalent of $435 dollars and forced to pay Sainsbury compensation for the defiled dairy.

Judge Not

From 1986 to 2003, it was a rainy night in Georgia for homosexuals who desired to engage in "deviant sexual intercourse" or "crimes against nature"—in other words, anal or oral sex. In 1986, the Supreme Court held that the federal right to privacy does not extend to sodomy. In *Bowers v. Hardwick,* Chief Justice Warren E. Burger cited the "ancient roots" of prohibitions against homosexual sex. It took the court seventeen years to realize that the long arm of the law shouldn't penetrate the bedroom of its citizens, and they overturned the ruling in 2003 with *Lawrence v. Texas,* 539 U.S. 558.

Tying the Knot

According to an October 31, 2002, article in the *Arizona Republic*, Mr. Rosaire Roy of Prince Albert, Saskatchewan, was sentenced to a year in jail for hiring someone to rob his store. Mr. Roy had arranged the robbery not to make money or collect insurance, but to fulfill a sexual fantasy: He had the robber force him to undress along with a female acquaintance because he dreamed of being tied up naked with her.

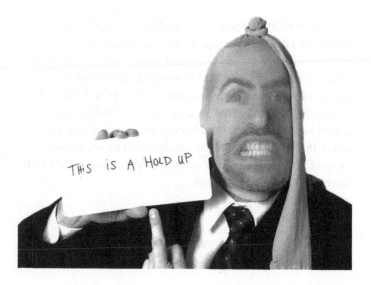

Deal Breakers

A woman in Hardwick, Georgia, filed for divorce, claiming that her husband, "stayed home too much and was much too affectionate."

A woman from Berlin, Germany, Heidi Berger, filed for divorce from her husband of sixty-nine years, Hans. In her divorce papers, she listed the cause of the divorce as "lack of sex." Heidi is 100 and Hans is 101.

Remember, Ladies First

Raquel Gonzalez, a twenty-four-year-old woman from Bradenton, Florida, was arrested and charged with felony domestic battery for beating up her boyfriend, thirty-year-old Esric Davis, by "hitting and scratching him, causing scratches near his eyes and nose," the police report read. According to a November 27, 2012, article in the *Daily Mail*, Gonzalez was outraged with Davis because he climaxed during intercourse and she didn't.

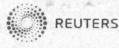

 REUTERS

February 6, 2002

Plenty of Sex Advised for Successful Pregnancy

A New Flame

"This is so embarrassing. We had never done that before, and now she's in the hospital, and my cat's dead!" exclaimed an unnamed man from New York City to the New York *Daily News* in 2005. While having sex, he and the woman he was with knocked over a candle that caught the comforter on fire. The flames quickly engulfed his entire apartment, injuring the woman and killing the cat.

"Because of the impropriety of entertaining guests of the opposite sex in the bedroom, it is suggested that the lobby be used for this purpose." —Actual sign in a Zurich hotel

One for the Casebook

In the landmark case, *United States v. Thomas*, in 1962, Navy Airmen Thomas and McClellan had been spending the night bar hopping. At one bar, McClellan was dancing with a highly intoxicated woman who passed out in his arms, and he and Thomas put the unconscious woman in McClellan's car. After a while, they thought it would be a good idea to rape the woman, and they both took turns. They then stopped at a gas station for help because the woman wasn't moving, and the attendant called the police, who discovered she was actually dead. The autopsy revealed that she had probably died while dancing. The two men tried to get out of the rape conviction by using the "impossibility" defense, claiming it's impossible to rape a dead person. They were found guilty of attempted rape because the court ruled that was their intention.

Behind Closed Doors

A twenty-three-year-old woman and a twenty-two-year-old man from Corona, New York, were discovered in his family's garage, nude and wrapped in a love embrace. Were his parents upset? No, they were horrified. According to a June 28, 2002, article in *Newsday*, the couple had kept the car running while they made out but forgot to open the garage door. By the time the boy's parents found the couple, they were already dead by carbon monoxide poisoning.

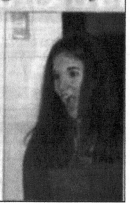

Student excited dad got head job

A Quack in the Case

A man was arrested on bestiality charges in New York's Hyde Park in the 1930s after being caught having sex with a duck. The man took his case to court and pleaded that, as a duck is a fowl and not a beast, he couldn't be charged with bestiality. He was acquitted.

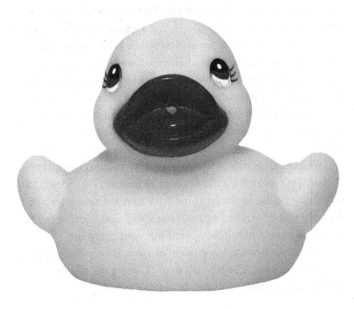

The Rules of Sex

With the enactment of the Disorderly Houses Amendment
Act of 1995, Australia legalized prostitution. Since it's legal, of
course, it has to be regulated, and that's where WorkCover, the
employee protection service of New South Wales, Australia,
comes in. They published guidelines for sex workers that warn,
among other things, about loose bed frames, unsanitary condi-
tions, sexually transmitted diseases, and, of course, repetitive
motion injuries. "A whole range of injuries can occur in the
workplace," a spokewoman said. "From slipping on a wet floor
in bathroom settings—because most brothels have an en suite
or bathroom attached to working rooms—to things like tripping
on stairs, slip hazards, a whole range of issues . . . the idea is to
make sure people in the [sex] industry have the resources to do
the right thing." According to a January 28, 2002, article in the
Weekly Standard, dim lighting may put your client in
the mood, but beware, the guidelines warn, it may also impair
your ability to see. The report's title? "Getting on Top of
Health and Safety."

Phone It In

A man from Bucharest, Romania, was feeling a little horny so
he thought he would use his phone to "reach out and touch
someone," so he called a telephone sex line. Sixty-two-year-old
Constantin Luican ran up a phone bill equaling $1,360. Was he
really that into the call? Actually, the reason he spent so much
time on the line is that he had fallen asleep. According to a
February 12, 2002, *Ananova* report, the Romanian pensioner
claimed he wouldn't pay the bill, which amounts to one year's
pay in Romania, because it was boring and he didn't have the
money. He was threatened with prison time if he refused to pay.

Blinded Me with Science

As an example of science catching up with what everyone already knows, a research study conducted in August 2002, using students from Glasgow University in Scotland, proved that members of the opposite sex become more attractive as one drinks more alcohol. The so-called "beer goggles" effect establishes that beauty may be more in the eye of the *beer holder* than in the eye of the beholder. Eighty students were shown color photographs and asked to grade the images' attractiveness while they consumed up to the equivalent of two-and-a-half glasses of wine. The study's leader, Professor Barry Jones from Glasgow University's psychology department, and Ben Jones from St. Andrews University, claimed the beer goggles effect is triggered when alcohol stimulates the nucleus accumbens, the part of the human brain that judges attractiveness.

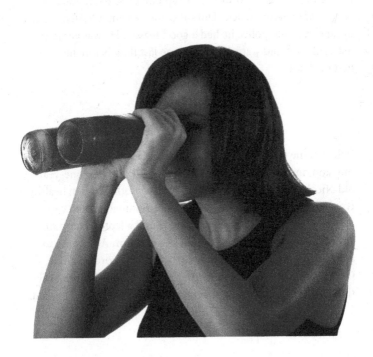

One for the Road

Twenty-four-year-old, Jeremiah Dubois was arrested and charged with rape according to a September 8, 2002, *Raleigh News and Observer* article. Dubois confessed and pleaded guilty to rape, but told police he had a good reason. He was getting married soon and wanted to have one last fling before he tied the knot.

Come and Go

Police in the town of Cirencester, located in southwestern England, investigated the unexpected death of thirty-one-year-old Nicola Paginton. The woman, who was otherwise in healthy condition, was found dead in her bed, presumably from cardiac arrest. Near her dead body they found a laptop computer with pornographic images, as well as a vibrator. According to a Fox News report from July 8, 2010, the local coroner, Alan Crickmore, ruled Paginton died of natural causes. "More likely than not this occurred from being in a state of arousal," he said.

When I Think of You, I Touch Myself

Nineteen-year-old Tina Rae Beavers of Great Falls, Montana, was arrested and charged with indecent exposure and unlawful communications with a prison inmate. Mrs. Beavers was taken into custody after she was seen writhing nude on the courthouse lawn, so that her husband, Ernie, could watch from his cell window. According to an October 6, 1996, article in the *Spokesman-Review*, Tina had been arrested for trying to smuggle cigarettes and marijuana to her husband.

Nothing to Balk At

A fifty-year-old Zambian man was so ashamed after being caught having sex that he hanged himself. According to a May 28, 2004, Reuters article, the man's wife heard strange noises coming from the house one day and discovered her husband having sex with a chicken. The man ran off in humiliation and later hanged himself. The chicken was slaughtered afterwards. Would have been less embarrassing if he had just been caught choking his chicken instead.

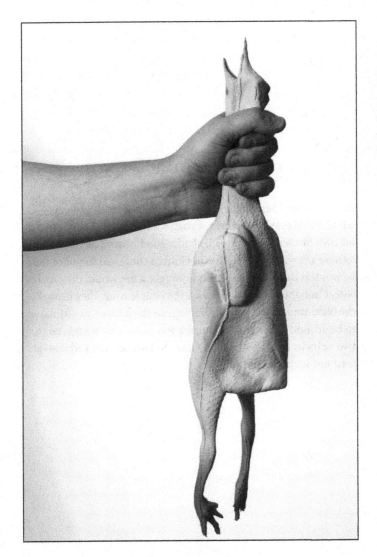

Burnin' Down the House

According to a September 12, 2003, *Ananova* article, a twenty-six-year-old man from Seget, Croatia, admitted he had set fire to his own house, but claimed he had a good reason; he didn't want to have sex with his wife. Svetin Gulisija confessed to police that he was too tired to have sex and thought a fire would distract his wife. Firefighters had to evacuate the couple while they brought the blaze under control. The damage to the house was estimated to be around $23,900, and Gulisija was ultimately sentenced to two years in jail. Now he won't have to have sex for a while—at least not with his wife.

Get Your Motor Running

A Cologne, Germany, court fined a man the equivalent of $795 dollars for hitting a road sign at sixty miles per hour while having sex. The man, who fled the scene, was later found and admitted he was having sex with a blonde hitchhiker who was straddling him while he drove. The twenty-three-year-old man was only charged for hit-and-run because there are no laws in Germany outlawing having sex while driving. Court spokesman Juergen Mannebeck said, "It's hard to believe but, in fact, no law was broken with the intercourse on the motorway. It's a situation lawmakers never thought about." According to a July 2, 2003, Reuters article, the man said he didn't know the identity of the woman, who left the scene naked.

Coitus Interruptus

While engaging in hot, steamy, passionate sex in a parked car near a reservoir in Denver, Colorado, a couple was spotted by a passing deputy. He wanted to make sure the sex was consensual and knocked on the steamed up window. The embarrassed couple gave the officer their identification and waited until he ran a quick background check. It turns out the man had an outstanding, unpayed fine for $63 for a dog-at-large charge. The officer requested payment of the fee and suggested the man keep it—the dog, I mean—on a leash from now on.

Two Balls and You're Out!

Gerald Allan Naud, a former pro boxer from Edmonton, Canada, pleaded guilty and was sentenced to twelve months in jail for sexual assault. Naud admitted to harassing a woman in an attempt to get her to kick him in the balls. The woman, who was unnamed, escaped his grasp and fled to her car. When she looked back, she noticed that Naud was frantically masturbating. According to a May 8, 2005, article in the *Canadian Press*, Naud first told police that he had made a $50 bet with a buddy that he wouldn't ask the woman to kick him in groin. "But there are no buddies, and the guy is a masochist," police Detective Wil Tonowski said.

Fashion Police

Baltimore's WBALTV reported on August 4, 2004, that Delaware state police responded to an outbreak of calls from complaining motorists about a man on the shoulder of I-95. They weren't concerned about his safety; they were concerned about what he was wearing, which was nothing but a woman's bra and panties on his head. Thirty-four-year-old Ronald Krischbaum was charged with misdemeanor exposure, lewdness, and resisting arrest.

I Go out Walking after Midnight . . .

According to an October 15, 2004, article in *New Scientist*, sleep medicine experts claimed to have successfully treated an Australian woman who suffered from an extremely rare sleep disorder: She screwed strangers while she was asleep. Like the more common sleep-talking and sleepwalking, someone suffering from sleep f**cking doesn't remember the event after she or he wakes up. The woman's husband brought this to her attention after he routinely found used condoms in their apartment that weren't his. One night, he discovered she had left the house. When he found her, she was having somnambular sex with another man. The doctor thought others who suffered from the same malady might not come forward because they were concerned their partners wouldn't really believe they "did it in their sleep."

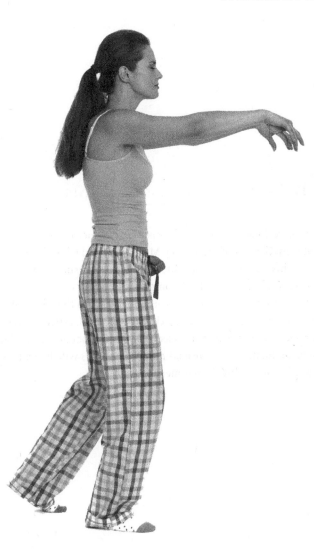

Paths of Righteousness for His Name's Sake

"I tried to follow the ways of Jesus," said former minister
Anthony Gifford of the Wesley Mimico United Church shortly
before his trial. Gifford admitted having consensual sex with
five adult members of the "moms and tots," but claimed he was
only counseling them so they could "get back to the basics of
Christianity." According to a February 12, 1998, article in the
Toronto Star, Gifford "counseled" the women aboard his yacht,
the Love Boat. Gifford also admitted he and his wife had a three-
way with one of his church members.

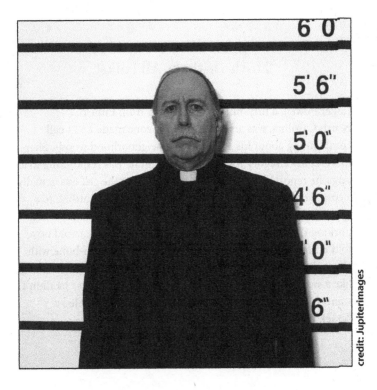

credit: Jupiterimages

Th-th-th-that's All Folks!

Roger Powell, a fifty-nine-year-old man from Enfield,
North Carolina, was arrested after someone made a 911 call
complaining about his activities in a neighborhood woods. Sheriff's Deputy Gregory Richardson thought he was responding to a
dog bite report, but was surprised to find out the call was actually
a complaint about Powell having sex with pigs. According to a
May 30, 2000, Reuters article, Richardson said he found Powell
porking the porker while talking to it. A local ten-year-old boy
told authorities that he had seen Powell playing ham-bone with
pigs at least three times. Powell explained that he had been acting
like a swine at least twice a day for the last year because he didn't
want to catch AIDS from his girlfriend, who he'd labeled a
"crack whore."

Sex, Lies, and Videotape

After being caught on a surveillance video stealing an undisclosed item from the police station, Constable Graham Hunt's attorney, Clayton Ruby, pointed out that Hunt had had an "expectation of privacy" while being in the room. In order to bolster his defense, Ruby divulged that later in the video a male officer was seen receiving oral sex from a female officer. According to an August 29, 2000, *Mount Carmel Daily Republican Register* article, Ruby insisted that had these two secret lovers not thought the room was beyond the reach of a surreptitious video, they wouldn't have felt safe to have sex.

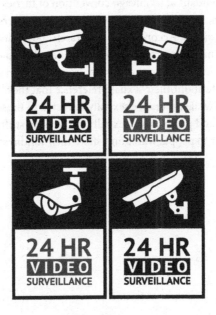

A Costume Ball

"If a (high school animal) mascot walked into a room surrounded by naked women, I'd be thinking about the mascot," said one attendant at a Chicago convention of furries (people, usually men, sexually obsessed with animal characters and animal costumes). According to the March 2001 edition of *Vanity Fair* magazine, more than four hundred people attended the convention, a majority of whom dressed as animals. Some are so passionate about their sexual preference that they "become" the animal, while others are sexually attracted to those who dress as animals, and plushies are sexually attracted to stuffed animals. Furries refer to people who don't share their fondness for fur as mundanes.

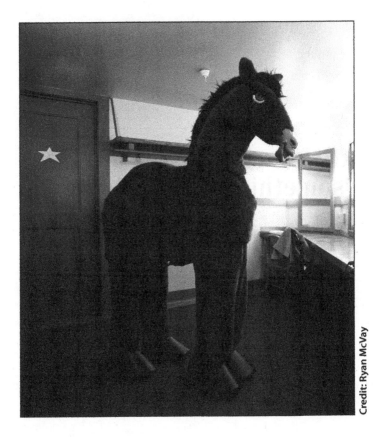

Credit: Ryan McVay

Girls' schools still offering 'something special' – head

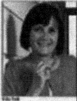

Get a Grip!

After the liquor began flowing at a house party, a British woman, Amanda Monti, made sexual advances to her former boyfriend, Geoffrey Jones, and his reaction was one he'll always regret—he rejected her. The jilted, and highly intoxicated, woman, violently wrestled with Jones, finally tearing his pants and underwear off and grabbing him by his jewels. She pulled so hard, she ripped off his left testicle. Not wanting to give back her newly plucked prize, the woman quickly hid it in her mouth. A friend of Jones was able to make the woman cough up the fur ball and he handed it back to the rightful owner saying, "that's yours." According to a January 11, 2005, article in the *Guardian*, Monti, although she couldn't remember the events of the night, pleaded guilty to unlawful wounding and was sentenced to two and a half years in jail. As for Jones, he won't be as nutty as he used to be, as doctors were unable to reattach his testicle.

All in the Family

Stacy Nihipali, from Cape Coral, Florida, was arrested after she and her thirteen-year-old daughter were caught breaking into a home, according to an August 30, 2001 *Associated Press* article. The home they broke into belonged to a man who refused to pay the mother/daughter team for sex. Prostitution was Nihipali's sole means of support and probably won't get her nominated for Mother of the Year.

So Good, It's Criminal

A neighbor of twenty-three-year-old Jamie Cheshire in East Sussex, England, called 999 (the English equivalent of 911) to report that she heard murderous screams coming from next door. Police were quickly dispatched and were met at the door by a towel-clad Mr. Cheshire. Cheshire told authorities that the screaming had been coming from his twenty-one-year-old girlfriend, Lenny Devaney. He told reporters, "We had been out to the pub and had two bottles of champagne and some tequila. We were sitting in the lounge and things got quite passionate. Lenny is a very passionate girl and a very loud one as well." The slightly-less-than-modest Lenny was quoted as saying, "It was hilarious. We were having sex in the living room and suddenly the police came round. They came in to see if I was all right but I was more than all right." According to a July 31, 2007, article in the *Sun*, Lenny also admitted, "I was probably making a lot of noise. He is a good lover."

A Streetcar Named Desire

The close quarters of a community theatre, the long hours together, and the feeling of partnership can provide the perfect breeding ground for a budding romance. But when fifty-three-year-old Jay Meisenhelder "fell in love" with a fellow actress, things weren't all rosy—mainly because the girl was sixteen years old. Meisenhelder wrote the young thespian an email stating, ". . . believe me, I know what love is. I love you as I have only loved two other women in my life." He persuaded the girl to meet him for a candlelit music session, where he served alcohol-free Banana Fosters and played the sound track from *The Phantom of the Opera*. Strangely enough, she asked him to take her home. Meisenhelder, who is married (or was when this story broke) claimed, "Nothing I did was illegal." Which is technically true, as Indiana state law defines an adult as anyone sixteen years or older. According to an April 13, 2007, article in the *Indianapolis Tribune Star*, when Meisenhelder's boss found out about the relationship, he was fired from his job—as the, get this, Deputy Prosecutor and Assistant Chief of the Sex Crimes Division. Meisenhelder insisted he was just "expressing a fantasy."

This is the same Meisenhelder who made news in 2002 when he successfully prosecuted a photographer for child exploitation and possession of child pornography for taking nude pictures of seventeen-year-old girls.

I Love Ewe

Students from Hawkeye Community College restrained Robert Allen Broderson from Waterloo, Iowa, after he was found in the school's hayloft early in the morning. Broderson wasn't alone in the loft, either. An October 27, 2000, Reuters article reported that in the corner of the loft was a bound ewe with her hindquarters elevated and a blue nightgown on the floor next to her. (Authorities weren't sure whether the nightgown was for Broderson or the ewe.) He was only charged with criminal trespass and animal abuse, as Iowa is one of twenty-six states that has no bestiality laws.

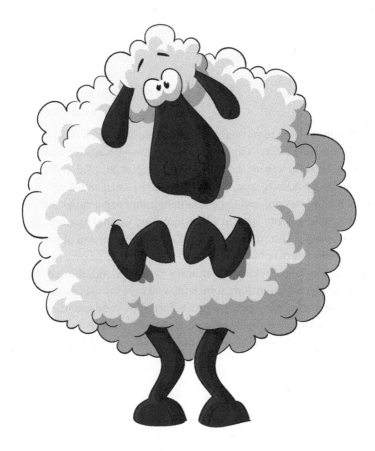

More Cowbells!

No one wanted to put eighty-one-year-old S. A. Balderson, of Richmond County, Virginia, out to pasture—because of what he does when he's there. According to an August 26, 2002, report on Fredericksburg.com, Balderson received a suspended sentence and was ordered to get counseling after being convicted of having sex with cows in a Westmoreland County pasture. Following up on complaints about Balderson's version of cow tipping, detective Merile Jones had set up a video camera in the field. The tape, provided by attorney Peggy Garland, showed the octogenarian making some milk shakes in his own particular style while wearing only a t-shirt, shoes, and sunglasses. Responding to the light sentence, Garland said, "What do you do with an eighty-something-year-old man who would do something like this?"

Hokey Pokey

Sodomy is defined as any non-penile/vaginal sex, including oral and anal sex. Innocent fun, right? You'd better beware where you do it. Even in the twenty-first century, you're in for more than a hot time if you're caught sodomizing anyone or anything in these states:

Misdemeanor: Alabama, Arizona, Arkansas, California, Kansas, Kentucky, Minnesota, Missouri, New York, Pennsylvania (married couples are exempt), Tennessee, Texas, Utah

Felony: District of Columbia (enacted 1892), Georgia, Idaho, Louisiana, Maryland, Massachusetts (enacted 1887), Michigan, Mississippi (enacted 1848), Montana, North Carolina (enacted 1868–69), Oklahoma, Rhode Island (enacted 1896), South Carolina (enacted 1902), Virginia

Public Displays of Affection

According to the *Miami News Times*, May and June of 2012 were good months for girl watching. Thirty-five-year-old Ashley Holton was arrested in May after she was discovered masturbating on the side of Highway 484 in Ocala, Florida. Less than a month later, on June 7, Tracy Mabb strutted into an intersection of South Dixie Highway in Pompano Beach, Florida, stripped off her clothes, and started masturbating.

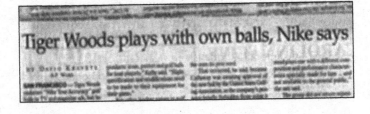

Tiger Woods plays with own balls, Nike says

A Shot in the Dark

A thirty-seven-year-old man from Helsinki, Finland, was sentenced to five years in prison for shooting the wife of his neighbor, who lived in the adjacent portion of a duplex. The man claims the woman, who arrived at his door wearing an open bathrobe, told him she had just put her son to bed and suggested the two of them have an evening drink. The two started fooling around, but their foreplay included a loaded gun. After a "shots fired" call, the police arrived at the residence and the man claimed the woman had shot herself. According to an October 31, 2001, Reuters article, when prosecutors asked the man why he needed a gun to get off, he claimed sex wasn't kinky without one.

Go Nuts for Doughnuts

Sandra McRae of Merrimack, New Hampshire, wanted to surprise a group of female temps on their last day working at Oxford Health Care so she stopped by Dunkin' Donuts and bought a box of Munchkins doughnut holes. According to a December 9, 1997, article in the *Sun Journal*, the women were not amused to find that more than a dozen or so of the sugary treats were shaped to form "a male sexual organ." McRae took the doughnuts to her boyfriend, who suggested she take them to the police (insert your favorite joke here). McRae filed a lawsuit against Dunkin' Donuts for "negligence and inflicting emotional distress." Glad they weren't cream filled.

Love is in Bloomers

The victim of an ongoing panty raid would have gotten her underwear in a knot over the theft—if she had any left. A woman in Oxford, Michigan, noticed that it wasn't her dryer that was stealing her panties. It was fifty-two-year-old Charles Dupon. Over a sixteen-year period, Dupon had routinely broken into the woman's house to steal her unmentionables. The woman's husband set up a video camera and caught Dupon with his hand in the panty jar and alerted police. According to an October 2, 1997, *Associated Press* article, police found 105 pairs of panties and other ladies' undergarments at Dupon's home. "This blows your mind," the woman said. "Out of 100 pairs of women's underpants, 90 were mine." The knickers nabber was charged with home invasion and faced up to twenty years in prison.

Indecent Exposure

What's a great name for a flasher? How about Jimmy Jewell? Well, Jewell picked the wrong person when he flashed his jewels in front of thirty-year-old Myko Kona. According to a May 31, 1997, article in the *Tuscaloosa News*, Kona was walking to work when Jewell pulled up in his van, asked her for directions, and then pulled out his pride and joy and started masturbating. Kona did some flashing herself. She pulled out her camera and took a picture of the little offender. "I pulled (the camera) up as soon as I could, and I just took the picture and he went ballistic," Kona said. "I thought at the time I had blown it." Jewell was arrested a few hours later and charged with indecent exposure and assault with a deadly weapon because he had attempted to run over Kona with his van.

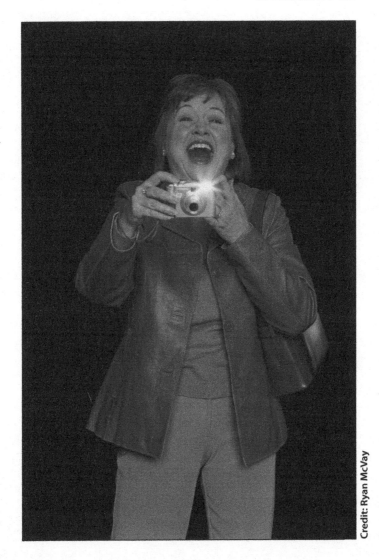

What's for Desert?

Everyone has heard that French waiters are rude, but the wait-staff at La Nouvelle Justine in New York's East Village might smack you on your ass—if you pay for it, of course. La Nouvelle opened in 1997 as the first S&M restaurant in New York, if not the world, and is filled with whip-toting mistresses, dog-collar-wearing busboys, BDSM paintings, and television monitors airing scantily clad women. In the March 2000 edition of *NY Rock*, the reviewer said, "Surprisingly, since La Nouvelle Justine is known more for its $20 spanking sessions than its culinary offerings, I found the food to be quite good." Manager Mistress Christine claimed, "At least one person from every table goes home realizing they like S&M. They buy paddles and chokers and collars and run around smacking their friends with it. It's more mainstream than people think."

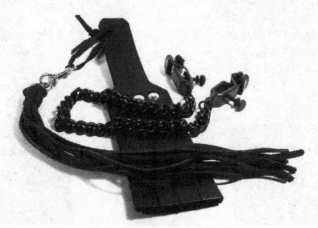

That Really Sucks!

Police and paramedics from Lakeland, Florida, were dispatched one morning by an emergency call made by a clerk at the Scottish Inn Motel. The clerk called at 4:45 a.m. and pleaded with the dispatcher to send help for a man who was stuck in the swimming pool. When the first responders arrived on the scene, they quickly ascertained what exactly was stuck: Robert Scott Cheuvront's penis. "As I approached the man," an officer reported, "I could see his pants were down to his knees and his penis was stuck in a suction hole located in the north side wall of the swimming pool." Even though the pool's pump had been shut off before police arrived, the man's member had swollen to such a degree that he couldn't remove it from the suction hole. According to a July 17, 1994, article in the *Daytona Beach News-Journal*, paramedics squeezed a lubricant into and around the suction fitting and were finally able to "free Willy" after about forty minutes.

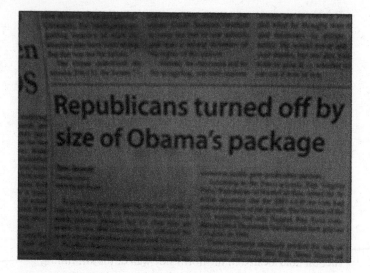

Republicans turned off by size of Obama's package

Saddle Up!

"I had a feeling he'd be back because I believe it's a compulsion-type thing with him," said horse owner, Allen McDearmid, about Patrick Louis Linn. McDearmid was talking about discovering, yet again, Linn having sex with one of his horses. According to an October 12, 2012, Huffington Post article, Linn, who was arrested in 2010 for naughty horseplay, was caught on video trespassing in the Tallahassee, Florida, stable. McDearmid said he knew there had been some horsing around because he noticed lubricant on the barn floor near Sunny the horse's stall.

What the Duck?

Police in Pattaya, Thailand, raided two bars and arrested four female go-go dancers and a man for performing a "hatching" sex show using live ducklings. According to a March 20, 1997, article in the *New Straits Times*, the baby ducks were placed in plastic eggs and inserted inside the dancers' vaginas. They would then be "hatched" on stage for the amusement of the audience. Surprisingly, there is no specific law against shoving live ducklings into a woman's vagina, and the dancers could only be fined $80 for performing immoral and improper acts.

A Real Knockout

A fifteen-year-old girl from Skokie, Illinois, pleaded guilty to assault after she "pummeled" her eighteen-year-old ex-boyfriend and blackened both of his eyes. According to a November 15, 2000, *Associated Press* article, the girl originally claimed the boy had tried to rape her but later recanted her story. She admitted she became enraged and attacked him after he refused to kiss her after the prom.

In Nieuwegein, The Netherlands, employees of a local stable became suspicious of some unstable activity after finding bales of hay and piles of stones forming a platform and placed behind several mares. Police arrested a twenty-one-year-old man who admitted "frequenting" several other animals in addition to the mares for the past month.

Feet, Do Your Duty

Police in Paramus, New Jersey, were putting their best foot forward trying to find a man who had a fetish for strange women's feet—or, to put it another way, a strange fetish for women's feet. According to a June 17, 1998, *Associated Press* article, Detective Kevin Smith said the suspect approached one woman while she was getting into her car outside Nordstrom's department store and pleaded with her to allow him to massage her feet. The other incident occurred a few minutes later when he snuck up on another woman from behind, grabbed her leg, knocked her into the front seat of her car, snatched off her right shoe, and tickled her foot, yelling, "You like it? Do you want more?"

Roll Tape

Contrary to popular belief, duct tape doesn't fix everything.
Just ask twenty-seven-year-old Randy Taylor of Adrian,
Michigan, who called 911 to report that he and his wife, Necoel,
had got caught up in a bondage game that led to her death.
When police arrived, they discovered that Necoel apparently
dead of asphyxiation with her mouth and nostrils covered
with duct tape. Taylor tried to explain that her death was
the result of a bizarre sex act but, "I doubt the prosecutor will
offer anything other than manslaughter," defense attorney
Jim Daley said.

An Unprincipled Principal

The old saying, "The principal is your pal" didn't hold true
in the case of fifty-five-year-old George S. Meadows, former
principal at Sylvia Elementary School in Beckley, West Virginia.
Meadows, who served as principal for seventeen years, was
arrested for soliciting prostitution. He wasn't soliciting a
prostitute, however. He was the prostitute . . . and he was in
drag. Meadows, who was wearing lipstick and a wig when he
was caught, tried to undercut the competition by offering the
undercover officers a lower price for oral sex. According to a
September 4, 1996, *Associated Press* article, Meadows, a father of
two sons, was suspended with pay from his principal position,
arrested on charges of prostitution, and fined $550 for a first
offense.

I'll Take a Stab at It

"Every night she asked me to make love to her three or four times and I couldn't take it any longer," said Chan Moon-sum. Moon-sum, a cook in Hong Kong, father of two, and a married man, was remarking on his arrest for stabbing his lover, Tsang Yim-lam. According to a June 5, 1996, Reuters article, Moon-sum was sentenced to three years in jail after admitting he stabbed his girlfriend because she demanded too much sex. Defense lawyer Andrew Macrae called Moon-sum "a man at the end of his tether."

Phoney Problem

Jose Aparecido Barbosa was finally caught after breaking into several stores over a series of months, but could only be arrested for breaking and entering and not burglary . . . because he never actually stole anything. According to a May 11, 1996, article in the *Manila Standard*, Barbosa broke into the various establishments so he could use their phone to call sex lines. "The guy is a pervert. He looks normal but a person like that can't be normal," a police spokesman said. Some stores were billed up to $20,000 per month because of Barbosa's fanatical phone fantasy fascination. The Rio Preto phone company made it known that the shop owners would not be charged for the phone calls.

Hello, Dolly!

Israel's Supreme Court denied the request of prison inmate, Amir Hazan, who petitioned the court for permission to have a sex doll in his cell. "I've been in jail since the age of fourteen. If they let me be with a woman, I would give up on getting a doll," said Hazan, who was serving a ten-year sentence for violent acts. According to a January 16, 1996, article in the Georgetown, Guyana, newspaper *Stabroek News*, the Prison Service argued they should be able to pull the plug on Hazan's request because having a sex doll could be used to fool prison guards in an escape attempt, hide drugs, or even cause inmates to fight over the doll.

I Can't Believe the Bride Wore White!

The village of Yeh Embang in the Jembrana regency of Bali, Indonesia, has a special punishment for people caught having sex with cattle—they make the perpetrator marry the cow. An eighteen-year-old man, identified only as GA, wore a traditional outfit during the wedding ceremony, and his bovine bride was draped in a white cloth. According to a June 15, 2010, article in the *Bali Times*, the cleansing ritual ceremony was to purify the man. What about the cow? Well, it was led into the sea and drowned.

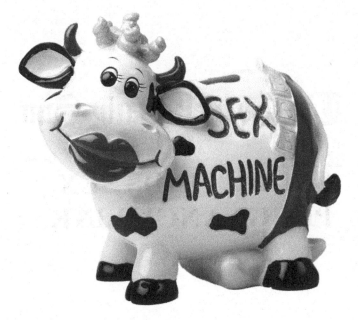

The Cornell Daily Sun

December 7, 1995

STUDY FINDS SEX, PREGNANCY LINK

A Piece of Ass

"Your worship, I only came to know I was being intimate with a donkey when I got arrested," said Sunday Moyo from Zvishavane, Zimbabwe, to the court magistrate in October 2011. According to a January 24, 2012, article in *New Zimbabwe*, the man claimed he was indulging in the services of a prostitute when she mysteriously transformed into the donkey he was caught violating.

Happy Endings

Going above and "beyond the call of duty," undercover council officials in England put it all on the line by visiting a massage parlor to make sure they weren't breaking the law. However, Labor Councilor Ben Summerskill questioned why they had to visit the same massage parlor seventeen times. According to a May 27, 1995, article in the *Moscow Times*, the inspectors defended their repetitive actions because although several scantily clad young women gave them "amateurish massages" before offering them sex, for a total of $3,160, they wanted to make sure it was the owner who was breaking the law and not the individual masseuses.

Blind Date Rape

A jury convicted Raymond Mitchell III, the "Fantasy Man" of Nashville, Tennessee, of rape by fraud and attempted rape by fraud by conning women into blindfolding themselves and then, alleging to be their boyfriend, convincing them to have sex with him. Prosecutors said that the majority of the women, purportedly hundreds of them, didn't fall for the ruse, thirty of them had encounters with Mitchell, and eight admitted they had sex with him. According to a June 20, 1996, *Associated Press* article, one woman confessed that she consented to have blindfolded sex twice a week over a two-month period and only stopped when she discovered Mitchell wasn't her boyfriend when the blindfold slipped off.

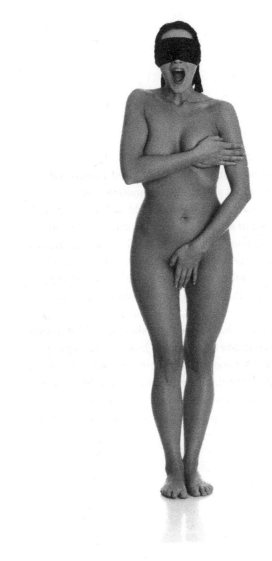

Eat My Shorts

Houston City Councilman Robb Todd received a complaint from a constituent about a store called Condoms & More and asked if he could do anything about it. Todd had the vice squad investigate the store to see if they were in violation of any ordinances but, it turned out, they weren't. But Todd was undaunted in his attempt to satisfy the one complainant, so he called out the city health inspector to see if the store had a license to sell the edible underwear they had on display. According to March 6, 1998, article in the *Avalanche-Journal Editorial*, the owner, Myrtle Freeman, didn't have a license so she just decided to stop selling the underwear. She did consider, however, paying the $200 annual permit fee and undergoing inspections so she could resume selling edible panties because she had some ideas to make them more appealing. "If we are going to go to all this trouble, I should at least heat them up," Freeman said. "If you want them fried or baked."

A Star is Born

Getting spotted by a talent scout is a dream that many an aspiring actor has. So when eighty-three-year-old Italian pensioner Spry Nilo Silvi was approached at a disco with his grandson and asked if he was interested in "making a film with beautiful young girls," he was flattered. According to a February 27, 1998, *Associated Press* article, Silvi said he was excited about starting his new career as a porn star. "For me it would be a pleasure," Silvi said. The octogenarian, who had been married twice and fathered six continued, "We talked about the possibility of filming some group scenes. I said I was willing, I'm not ashamed at all." He did, however, have some restrictions on what he was willing to do. "I won't use a condom because, at my age, I could have some problems with it. I prefer doing it without, the old-fashioned way." Asked by a reporter whether he worried about AIDS, Silvi added, "I'm old, but I'm not stupid. They've told me they are all young, healthy girls. Anyway AIDS takes ten years to develop. I'll die first."

One Lump or Two?

The people in the sleepy little town of Selby, South Dakota, with a population of only seven hundred, made the news in 1995 when a man impersonating a Medicare worker convinced two elderly women to allow him to perform a breast exam on them. According to a November 3, 1995, article in the *Orlando Sentinel*, the man showed up at their apartments and separately told the two women (aged eighty and ninety-two) that he routinely did free breast exams. The two women consented to the exam, but got suspicious when, after fondling their boobs, he quickly left and drove away in a red sports car.

You Don't Get Jack

Obviously fifty-two-year-old Mehmet Esirgen of Ankara, Turkey, suffered from penis envy and had every intention to do something about it. According to a February 22, 1997, article in the *Moscow Times*, Esirgen's own son shot him in the leg because of his insistence on having a penis transplant from a donkey. This wasn't the first time he wanted to be hung like a mule, either. On two previous occasions, Esirgen purchased two donkeys, cut off their penises, and appealed to doctors to perform the penile transplant, which they refused to do. His family thought Esirgen was a jackass for his failed attempts, but he claimed that he needed the donkey dongs to cure his sexual impotence. Although Esirgen didn't get his wish, he threatened to buy a fourth donkey as soon as he recovered from his leg wound.

Taking a Bite out of Crime

For two years, police in Jakarta, Indonesia, had been on the lookout for the infamous "penis biter." After receiving complaints from at least five young schoolboys who had their penises bitten by the mystery woman, police finally found the perpetrator at a bus terminal in Kupang, on the western half of Timor Island. According to a June 5, 1996, article in the *Irish Times*, police were alerted to the penis biter's whereabouts when a bus driver was heard screaming in pain. After the biter was arrested, authorities were surprised to find out he had a penis of his own. The penis biter was actually a man dressed in drag.

An Illuminating Idea

"Stick it up your ass" might as well have been the report published in the November 1982 issue of *Annals of Emergency Medicine*. The title of the report was "Removal of 100-Watt Electric Bulb from Rectum." The report started with a short list of confirmed items that had been removed from the rectum of patients: "stones, coke bottles, plastic vibrators, pencils, sticks, a baseball, knives, screwdrivers, the U-bend of a sink, a sponge rubber ball, glass tumblers, a pickle bottle, and a beer glass. This case report adds to the list a 100-watt electric bulb, an object not previously reported. . . ." A fifty-four-year-old man admitted he had gotten drunk and accepted a $100 bet to insert a light bulb into his rectum. He thought the bulb would be easy to remove, but was unable to get it out. After two days, he began having difficulty defecating and urinating. A rectal examination revealed "a hard, smooth, globular mass." Doctors weren't sure if the man actually had a light bulb up his butt or if his colon had a bright idea.

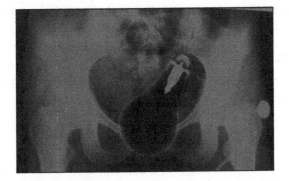

Cheaters by Country

According to a 2011 survey conducted by the condom manufacturer Durex, Nigerian women are the most unfaithful in the world at 62 percent, followed by Thai women (59 percent), Malaysian women (39 percent), and Russian women (33 percent). Thai men get the gold medal for cheating (54 percent), South Korean men the silver (34 percent), and Malaysian men the bronze (33 percent). As reported in a December 7, 2011, article in the *Daily Times*, 29,000 people in 36 countries were interviewed for the report.

It's the Thought that Counts

The English town of Bournemouth became concerned about child sex abuse and wanted to raise awareness that it could happen anywhere, not just in the notorious sex-tourist spots. According to a February 27, 1997, article in the *Brand Republic News*, a public service campaign was created by the Children's Society and their slogan, emblazoned on billboards across the town, was, "Why travel 6,000 miles to have sex with children when you can do it in Bournemouth?"

Man's Best Friend

Police were dogging forty-nine-year-old Bradley Brainard, of Atascadero, California, for suspicion of selling drugs to prison inmates when they came across something that got them barking up another tree. While searching Brainard's home, police discovered a video of the plumber "on a bed, naked, wearing a woman's brassiere along with a chocolate Labrador" with which he was performing various sexual acts, according to an arrest warrant quoted in the December 31, 2009 edition of the *San Luis Obispo Tribune.* The article quoted Brainard as saying, "It's something I got into that I never should have gotten into."

Mom of the Year

Thirty-year-old Deborah Lee Towe of Anderson, California, admitted to having sex with her fifteen-year-old daughter's friends at her home, in a Walmart parking lot, and even in an elementary school parking lot. Towe told authorities, "I felt young. I missed all those years," according to September 19, 2009, Redding.com article. She claimed the reason she had sex with several young boys (some as young as fifteen) was so they wouldn't try to have sex with her daughter. She was sentenced to a year in jail and five years' probation.

REUTERS

January 1, 2002

You Can't Buy Love,
but Euro Brings
Cheaper Sex

Three's Company

A lot of people fantasize about having a three-way, but fifty-one-year-old George Bartusek was about to have a three-way of a different kind when he was caught having sex in the parking lot of a Publix market with two blow-up dolls. "As I walked by, I saw this guy with two blow-up dolls kissing them and bouncing them and trying to get people's attention," a witness told WPDB-TV. Other than the two dolls in the front seat, police discovered a pack of king size Pall Mall Menthol cigarettes and three packages of Reese's Peanut Butter Cups. At least Bartusek brought enough to share.

Eureka!!!!

Apparently, Jason Leroy Savage had been on too many dates that just blew and wanted a surefire date that would really suck. According to a March 26, 2009, *Associated Press* article, Savage was arrested and sentenced to ninety days in jail after police caught him having sex with a car wash vacuum. The twenty-nine-year-old was found priming the pump at a Detroit car wash and eventually pleaded no contest to indecent exposure. Unfortunately, the article didn't specify the type of air-freshener he chose.

Nothing to Sneeze At

In an April 18, 2008, report by *ABC News Medical Unit*,
"[A] person with a sneeze fetish can find erotic pleasure in
those few seconds" when "the eyes close as the body prepares
to forcefully expel air," but "experts are stumped as to why."
As with any sexual deviation, there's at least one Internet site
dedicated to it, and sneeze fetishism is no exception. "She
has the cutest sneeze ever," said one member of an Internet
"sneeze fetish forum." Others on the forum reminisce about
previous sneeze (or sternutation) experiences. One member
remembered the high he experienced when he discovered that
his college roommate had allergies and would be constantly
sneezing.

Getting Benched

Now, here is a guy who was really into knotty sex. Hong Kong police and medical personnel were dispatched to Lan Tian Park to assist a man who was stuck after trying to have sex with a park bench. Forty-one-year-old Le Xing, who was described as a "lonely and disturbed" man, said he thought it would be fun to have sex with the bench. Reports described in an August 12, 2008, article in the *Telegraph* say that medical personnel tried to relieve the swelling by removing some of Xing's blood, but eventually had to cut the bench from the ground and take it, with Xing attached, to a city hospital.

The Object of Her Affection

With a name like Erika La Tour Eiffel, one would think that she'd be related, somehow, to the man who created the Eiffel Tower. Well, she's actually the tower's wife. The thirty-seven-year-old woman is one of a handful of people in the world called objectum sexuals—people who fall in love with inanimate objects. She changed her last name when she married the Tower. She had been married before, according to a March 9, 2009, article in New York *Daily News*, first to Lance, a bow that helped her become a world-class archer. Then she fell in love with the Berlin Wall. She even had a fling with a piece of fence she keeps in her bedroom.

Wall of Shame

Another case of objectum-sexuality involved Eija-Riitta Berliner-Mauer, whose surname means "Berlin Wall" in German. Berliner-Mauer, who lives in Liden, northern Sweden, married the graffiti-covered concrete wall in 1979. "I find long, slim things with horizontal lines very sexy," Berliner-Mauer told the *Telegraph* in 2008. "The Great Wall of China's attractive, but he's too thick—my husband is sexier." I guess this makes her a real bricklayer.

Nuts, Bolts, and Screws

According to an article in the June 1, 2008, edition of the *Daily Telegraph*, doctors at Hornsby Hospital in Sydney, Australia, were surprised to see a man brought in by a fire rescue crew who had gone nuts over washers. The fire rescue crew was unable to help the man remove the sixteen stainless steel washers he had around his penis and was forced to take him to a surgeon. The unnamed man underwent a ninety-minute procedure to have the washers removed with no damage to his manhood except for "damage maybe to his pride."

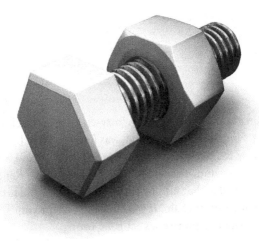

"E" for Effort

An enterprising pervert, forty-year-old Michael Derenberger, of Hernando, Florida, was charged with "Loitering or Prowling" on June 2, 2006. Derenberger was caught placing a long pole with a hook attached to the end through a bedroom window to pull down the comforter of a young girl as she slept.

According to the *Daily Record*, a forty-eight-year-old church organist from Stockton, England, was found dead in his home on January 26, 2007. He was naked, and his hands and feet were bound to a vacuum cleaner. Police reported that Ian Kemp's legs were "tied at the shins by brown parcel tape" and his wrists bound with a silver chain. It was concluded that Kemp's death was the result of a bizarre sex act gone wrong.

Getting the Finger

The New York *Daily News* reported on November 3, 2012, that twenty-nine-year-old Jennifer Piranian must have wanted a little more cream in her coffee after she was discovered masturbating at a Starbucks in Bradenton, Florida. "No one could ever say for sure what she was doing, and I'm pretty sure the video didn't show anything definitive. But her hands went into her pants when she was wigging out," Bradenton Police spokesman Josh Cramer said. The arresting officer received permission from Piranian to search her purse, at which time he discovered "a glass stem" pipe that contained cocaine residue. She was caught red-handed and arrested for possession of narcotics and drug paraphernalia.

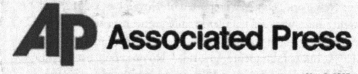

Associated Press

May 3, 2007

'Giggles The Clown' Jailed On Sex Charges

You Big Baby

Workers at a daycare center in Brookfield, Wisconsin, heard someone pounding on their back door and just assumed it was an impatient parent. But to their surprise, when they opened the door, they saw twenty-year-old Lance A. Binkowski, dressed in large footie pajamas, sucking on a pacifier, and holding a teddy bear and a diaper bag. According to a November 20, 1993, article in the *Milwaukee Sentinel*, Binkowski was soon arrested and charged with reckless endangerment after he ran from police. The chief of police stated that Binkowski "had his own personal reasons" for being there, but intended no harm to the children. Binkowski obviously suffered from paraphilic infantilism (see the Deviant Dictionary on page 199).

Just Like Falling off a Bicycle

"In almost four decades in the law, I thought I had come across every perversion known to mankind," said Sheriff Colin Miller. "But this is a new one to me. I have never heard of a 'cycle-sexualist.'" Miller was talking about Scot Robert Stewart of Ayr, Scotland, who was caught by two cleaning women frantically pumping his bicycle, in bed. The fifty-one-year-old was wearing only a shirt, said Miller, and when the two women opened the door, he exclaimed, "What is it, hen?" before continuing to "move his hips back and forth as if to simulate sex." According to a November 14, 2007, article in the *Telegraph*, Stewart was put on probation for three years as well as on the sex offenders list.

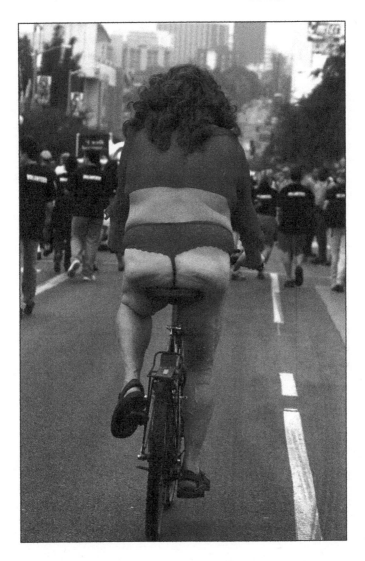

Come Together, Right Now

According to a 2012 survey conducted by the condom maker Durex, nearly half (46 percent) of the one thousand American adults ages eighteen and older questioned between March 16 and March 22, 2012, responded that they're more likely to see Big Foot than "finish" at the same time as their partner. The survey also uncovered that 37 percent admitted that sex ends too quickly while 14 percent revealed that sex lasts longer than they would like.

Locking up the Jewels

Reuters reported in February 1994 that a serial flasher had been showing his goods in Adelaide, Australia, since April 1992 and had given more than fifty victims an eye-full. Flashers are nothing new, but this male perpetrator had the lock on weirdness. For reasons unknown, the flasher was routinely identified by the padlock he always wore around his genitals.

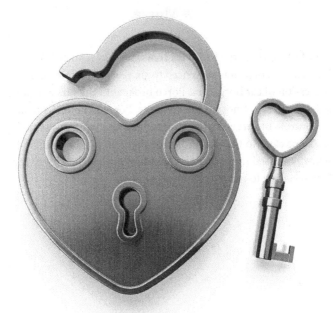

Keep Your Hands to Yourself

The New York *Daily News* reported on October 28, 1993, about the trial of New York City Correction Department doctor Jerzy Gajewski, who was accused of fondling a woman in a subway station the previous year. But before a verdict could be reached, Gajewski was suspended without pay after he allegedly fondled the court stenographer.

A Murse

On May 23, 1995, the *Knoxville News-Sentinel* reported that Stephen N. Porco was sentenced to six years in prison for a succession of car burglaries. Porco broke into the cars and stole lady's purses, but not for the contents. Porco suffered from an uncontrollable urge to gratify himself using a women's handbag. A source close to the case projected that Porco had stolen and sexually abused more than five hundred purses, thereby giving new meaning to the term "purse snatcher."

A Real Blow-Hard

Twenty-year-old Shawn George thought he had a foolproof way of getting women to talk to him, but the only proof was that he was the fool. George was arrested in Syracuse, New York, according to an April 21, 1996, *Edmonton Journal* article, for calling various female office employees (approximately one hundred women in thirty different buildings) and requested responses to a sexually explicit and phony questionnaire. If they refused, he threatened to blow up their buildings.

Leaving a Tip

An article in the February 1996 issue of the journal *Genitourinary Medicine*, which covers issues related to genital and urinary organs, reported the case of a man who was prescribed surgery stemming from complaints of genital pain. The embarrassed man hesitantly admitted to physicians that, while engaging in sex with his wife approximately twelve years previous, she had inserted a mascara brush into his urethral opening. Doctors discovered the tip of the brush had broken off and that fibrous tissue had grown around it, causing the man severe pain.

Screw It!

Traditionally, *fornication* refers to consensual sexual intercourse between two people not married to each other. Believe it or not, there are still states that have laws against fornication:

Arizona (misdemeanor)

District of Columbia (misdemeanor)

Florida (misdemeanor, enacted in 1868)

Georgia (misdemeanor, enacted in 1833)

Idaho (misdemeanor)

Illinois (misdemeanor)

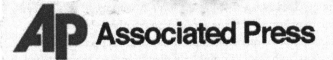

Associated Press

December 11, 2008

Man handcuffs his wife to the bed, loses key

Paging Dr. Scholls

David Donathon of Medina, Ohio, went through counseling and was even imprisoned for his fetish for smelly feet. According to a January 15, 1999, article in the *Orlando Sentinel*, he was headed back to prison after being arrested on telephone harassment charges. Apparently Donathon couldn't always get his foot in the door, so he would simply call people and ask them if their feet stank. Donathon's lawyer, Michael Westerhaus, claimed his client could benefit from an intensive program for sex offenders, even though he'd been in several before. "He realizes what he does is wrong, but he is unable to stop himself," Westerhaus said.

In St. Paul, Minnesota, John O. Sexton, was arrested for cutting off fifty strands of a woman's ponytail and sentenced to forty-five-days in jail. According to an August 27, 1998 article in the *Duluth News-Tribune*, Sexton offered to pay for the woman's hair but was rejected, after which he snipped them and ran. Following his arrest, he apologized for his sexual "urges about hair" and promised to seek counseling.

There's No Place Like Home

Jeffery Marriott, a fifty-year-old resident of Port St. Lucie, Florida, was arrested after a witness called police complaining that the man was masturbating in his own front yard and "working real hard." The unidentified witness claims he saw Marriott "walking back and forth masturbating in the driveway, the front yard, and between the trucks" parked in front of his home. According to a June 12, 2012, article in the *Miami News Times*, when police arrived they discovered an "unknown clear liquid substance" on his doorknob.

Give That Man a Hand!

It's usually an insult when someone gives you the finger, but for thirty-eight-year-old Richard Lee Sanders, it gets him off. Sanders was charged with three counts of disorderly conduct for sucking the fingers of women in Burnsville and Apple Valley, Minnesota. Burnsville prosecutor Michael Mayer stated that Sander's situation was "his weirdest case in his sixteen years on the job." According to July 14, 2001, article in the *St. Paul Pioneer Planet*, Sanders was charged with the same offense the month before. His modus operandi was to approach women, compliment them on how attractive their fingernails were, and then quickly stuck them in his mouth and suck on them.

His Heart's Ablaze

Some people love drama in their lives; in some cases, they love it so much, they get off on it. According to a June 5, 2002, *Ananova* article, police in Thailand arrested a man for a setting a series of vehicular fires. At first, the man claimed that he had done this as a way to relieve stress. However, after questioning, he confessed that he got a sexual thrill from setting the fire and drinking beer while the police and firemen came to put it out. The unnamed man had already served two years in prison for a similar offense and after his release . . . he became a volunteer firefighter.

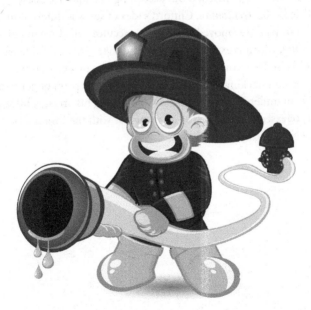

Ah, Nuts!

In Bucks County, Pennsylvania, twenty-seven-year-old Brandon Clifford pled guilty to attempting to sexually entice an underage girl by use of the Internet. But according to a May 10, 2001, article in the *Trentonian*, Clifford's idea of sex was different than most others. He enjoyed what the prosecutor called Asian Ball Busting, which is exactly what it sounds like. The painful fetish could also be accomplished, according to the prosecutor, by someone smacking Clifford's scrotum with the palm of her hand with an underneath striking blow. Following his arrest, Clifford was released from his job as an inspector with the Immigration and Naturalization Service.

One-Armed Bandit

According to a June 16, 2001, article in the *Dallas Morning News*, police were still no closer in finding a man who had attacked thirteen women over the past year. The unknown assailant would approach women and then either bite or lick their arms and then run away.

Sex . . . It's What's for Dinner

They're called Splosher parties, and they're becoming popular
nationwide, especially (and not surprisingly) in San Francisco. A
2002 article in *SF Weekly* expounded on this quasi-sexual fetish
in which people roll around and wallow, semi-nude, in globs
of cream, mud, soups, syrups, cakes, pies, or anything icky and
sticky. One couple highlighted in the article took this to another
level. The woman role-played being a customer at a restaurant,
and the man a clumsy waiter who continually spilled food on
her—all to her delight.

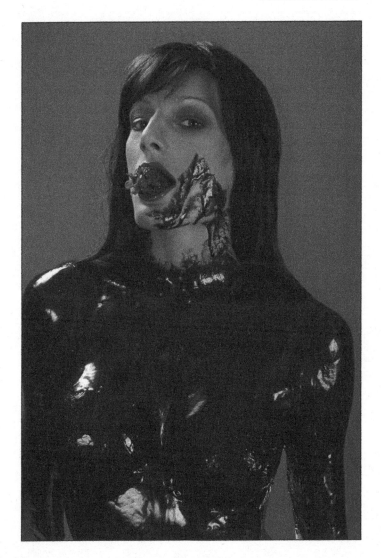

Jacket Off!

The Canadian newspaper *Sault Star* reported on the weird fetish of fifty-eight-year-old Gerard Lancop, who was sentenced to nearly two years in prison for harassment and nuisance. Lancop has what his psychiatrist describes as a fetish for women's coats. After his arrest, approximately 236 coats were found in Lancop's home. This guy needs to keep his sexual perversions under wraps.

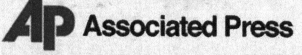

Associated Press

February 28, 2009

Necrophilia charges mount for former morgue worker already serving sentence for sex with corpse

Nappy Nabber

Deputies from Orange County, North Carolina, charged
Jason Glen Humphrey with taking indecent liberties, assault
on a female, assault on a child under twelve years old, and assault
by a show of violence and breaking into a motor vehicle.
So, what was this bad man after? Soiled diapers. According to a
July 29, 2003, article in the *Herald-Sun*, the twenty-nine-year-old
man was arrested after a year-long spree of leering at mothers
as they changed their baby's poopy diapers. This time, he
reached into a car at a car wash and attempted to take the
toddler's dirty diaper and was arrested. He was being held
under $200,000 bond.

You Show Me Yours

To crack a "pedophile ring," police officer James Marriner requested confidential sexual histories, pubic hair samples, and nude photos from members of the small Bible-based community he lived in near Ipswich, Queensland, in Australia. However, according to a September 23, 2003, article in the *New Interactive*, there was no "pedophile ring," and Marriner requested and received the abovementioned items for his own sexual gratification. He was arrested and charged with fifteen counts related to sexual harassment.

Dream Catcher

The *Baton Rouge Advocate* reported on September 30, 2003, that twenty-four-year-old Steve Danos was arrested after allegedly sneaking into young women's apartments. Danos didn't sexually abuse the women; he merely snuggled with them and occasionally folded their laundry while they slept.

Dental Damn!

Thirty-nine-year-old Masafumi Natsukawa was arrested in Yokohama, Japan, for tricking more than thirty young girls, according to a January 18, 2006, article in the *Mainichi Daily News*. Apparently, Natsukawafor convinced the girls to open their mouths under the ruse of checking them for tooth decay. When they opened wide . . . he licked their tongues.

Toeing the Line

Michael Codde, a former schoolteacher, was sentenced in Santa Cruz, California, to a year in jail on charges of felony child molestation. According to a January 29, 2006, article in the *San Jose Mercury News*, several teenage boys came forward and accused the forty-four-year-old Codde of putting whipped cream on their toes and watching them lick it off while he took photographs.

The bra celebrates a pair of historic milestones this year

After 100 years of innovation, the device still holds up

By SHARON FINK
St. Petersburg Times

It's time to mark two important milestones in the bra, the Wonderbra, the water bra, bras are constantly evolving

Although it often may not feel like it, the industry's No. 1 goal is comfort, said Norah Alberto, senior style director at Maidenform.

"You kind of want to forget you're wearing (a bra)," she moment that got the cultural pot stirrer as much attention for her image as her music.

Bras as outerwear were eventually joined by bustiers and corset tops (without bones in them). Then slips started being worn as dresses. Camisoles became a dressier kind of tank top. And under-

Judge Not!

If you were to ask former Oklahoma district judge Donald Thompson if anything was worn under his robe, he would probably answer, "No, everything is in perfect working order." Thompson was charged with indecency and finally scheduled for arraignment according to a January 4, 2006, segment on Court TV. Twelve months earlier, the judge was charged for allegedly using a noisy masturbation aid during trials and other court business. He was also charged with another count of indecency based on a court reporter's accusation that she observed him shaving his pubic hair during a trial.

Water Sports

Leave it to the Russians to come up with a weird sport: water rafting on inflatable sex dolls. According to a 2006 article in the *Moscow News*, forty-year-old Igor Osipov was disqualified from the rafting tournament held on the Vuoksa River near St. Petersburg, Russia, after spectators "saw signs of recent sexual activity on (Osipov)'s doll."

Unbridled Passion

Alfred Thomas Steven had an unstable fantasy about horses. The sixty-nine-year-old eventually was arrested in the La Purisma Mission Park in Lompoc, California, according to a September 9, 2006 report on KSBY-TV. Apparently, to satisfy a longtime fantasy, Steven poured olive oil all over his body, covered himself in oats, and laid down so the horse would nibble and lick the grain off him.

Getting a Foot Up

An eighty-year-old woman in Perry, Georgia, reported that while she was at the local Wal-Mart, a man approached her and asked for her help in satisfying his "religious" ritual. According to a September 9, 2006, article in the *Macon Telegraph*, the man, who was sitting on the floor of an aisle, asked the woman to step on his hands and spit on him, which she did. But when he began to lick her feet, she reported him.

Fill This Out

If a man claiming to be a recruiter for T-Mobile requests a urine sample to complete your employment application, don't do it. But that's just what happened to two women who submitted their samples to thirty-six-year-old Kevin Oliver, in Omaha, Nebraska. According to a February 1, 2007, report by MSNBC, Oliver was arrested and convicted of criminal impersonation.

Dummy Lover

Ronald Dotson suffers from a sexual perversion called statuephilia, which is a strong sexual attraction to statues, mannequins, life-size dolls, etc. The thirty-nine-year-old didn't pay for his "dates," however. He stole them. "I thought I was getting my life together," he told the judge after he pled no contest to his seventh statuephilia-related offense in thirteen years. According to a January 26, 2007, *Detroit Free Press* article, Dotson attempted to break into a Ferndale, Michigan, store to steal a mannequin outfitted in a French maid's uniform. His previous arrests were for stealing a mannequin in a pink dress and bobbed hair, and in another case he was found in an alley with three mannequins wearing lingerie.

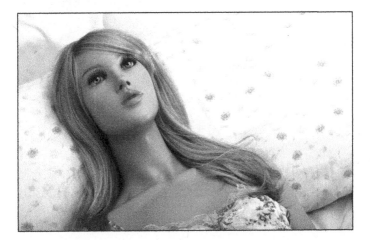

Writing a Wrong

Frank Ranieri was arrested in New York City and charged with impersonating a police officer. Did Ranieri try to extort money from peoples or falsely arrest them? No. What the twenty-five-year-old was convicted of was a particular deviancy called paraphilia or piquerism. According to a June 7, 2007, article in the *New York Post*, the man tried to bribe teenage girls to let him stab them in the buttocks with a ball-point pen.

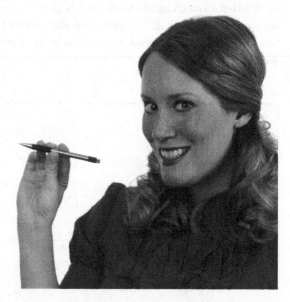

Sign, Sign, Everywhere a Sign

Sexual deviancy is everywhere, but sixty-year-old Verle Dills showed that extreme weirdness is just a sign of the times. According to an August 1, 2007, article in the *Sioux Falls Argus Leader*, Dills was arrested after authorities discovered a number of homemade videos showing Dills having sex in public with traffic signs.

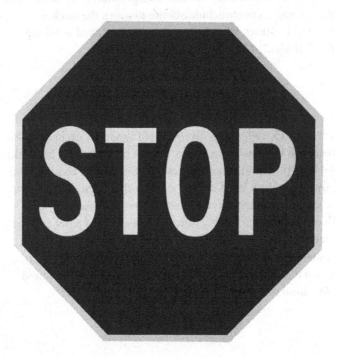

Tiny Bubble

Jeff Doland of Uniontown, Ohio, reached a new level of weird when he was arrested during an Internet sting. According to a July 27, 2007, article in the *Canton Repository*, authorities set up an operation to convince Doland to fly to Miami under the assumption that he was going to meet a "mother" who would allow him to take photographs of her two adolescent daughters while she dunked them underwater. Doland admitted that he had an overwhelming desire to watch the mother pretend to drown her daughters because he "liked watching the bubbles."

Dog-Day Afternoon

On April 15, 1997, thirty-five-year-old Sandra L. Archer was sentenced to the maximum of two years in jail in Omaha, Nebraska for cruelty to animals and one count of disorderly conduct. Her boyfriend, Mark W. Williams, was also charged with six counts of cruelty to animals, assault and battery, and disorderly conduct. Police investigated a disturbance call, and Archer said the argument was about returning several videotapes. The videos contained footage of Archer and Williams having sex atop a group of dogs (some very ill) and rabbits the couple acquired from local shelters.

Crime and Punishment

In August 1997, Malaysia's Johor Baru Religious Affairs Department announced that sexual "deviants" convicted of a crime would from now on not only serve time in prison—they would also be bound and whipped.

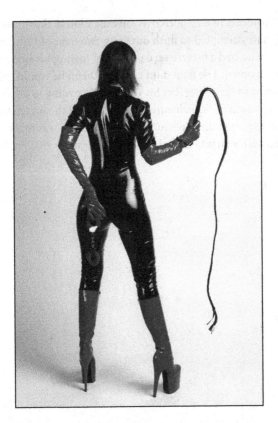

Spit Take

Female officers in an undercover investigation in downtown Cincinnati attempted to flush out forty-two-year old Anthony Searles, who had a bizarre sexual fetish of tossing his spit on well-dressed women. The man didn't spit on them; he would spit in his hand and then fling it at his victims. According to a July 19, 2001, article in the *Cincinnati Enquirer*, one of the undercover officers expected the expectorator, and after she was marked as his next saliva target, she quickly arrested him.

Hair Today, Gone Tomorrow

Mark Philip Thackery approached the mother of a seven-year-old girl with long hair at a garage sale and offered her $100 for the girl's ponytail. According to an April 16, 1999, article in the *Spartanburg Herald-Journal*, the mother told the forty-six-year-old man to leave, but he was seen at least seven times later parked near the family's home. On April 7, 1999, the girl's father spotted Thackery apparently trying to break into the family home to steal hair-related items and confronted him.
Later that evening, police found Thackery and arrested him for stalking a minor and attempted home invasion and placed him in jail on a $100,000 bond.

If This Boat Is Rockin'

According to an article in the *San Francisco Chronicle*, Sausalito, California, school board member Cathomas Starbird was sentenced to fifteen days in jail for assaulting a female friend aboard the Starbirds' houseboat in 1999. After a birthday dinner for her husband, Mrs. Starbird wanted her friend to "blow out" her husband's candle. When the woman refused to orally pleasure the birthday boy, Starbird became furious, jumped on her friend, and bit her on the face.

She's All Talk

Kire Iliovski, a twenty-five-year-old man from Prilep, Macedonia, talked on the phone for more than 135 hours to an extremely friendly and provocative woman he thought could be his perfect future bride. When he received a phone bill for $15,322, Iliovski made an official complaint to his local phone company, Macedonian Telecommunications, to have the bill forgiven. Iliovski told local media, as reported by *Ananova* on November 20, 2003, "I couldn't believe my eyes when I saw the bill. I thought I was calling an agency for possible marriage connections, not a sex line."

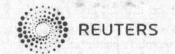

REUTERS

January 25, 2001

Man on Way to Brothel Finds Wife Working

Like a Puppet on a String

I'm sure most of you have heard of sock puppets, but what about a cock puppet? Well, forty-four-year-old Timothy Wayne Martin, of Auburn, Washington, was arrested after witnesses saw him using his genitals as a marionette. Martin was seen sitting partially with a string tied around his penis. According to police who arrested Martin at the Arcadia Apartment Complex, he "was apparently manipulating it with the string like a puppet." An article in the May 29, 2009, edition of *Metro* (UK) stated that police also discovered Martin was in possession of a small amount of methamphetamine and a pornographic magazine. He was sent to the Norm Maleng Regional Justice Center in Kent on $25,000 bail and probably wound up as someone's meat puppet there.

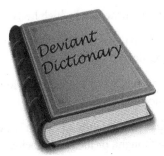

Abasiophilia: A psychosexual attraction to people with impaired mobility (spinal braces, crutches, neck braces, wheelchairs, leg braces, etc). There is a subset known as a cast fetish.

Acomocliticism: A fetish for a sexual partner having hairless genitals.

Acrotomophilia: A paraphilia (a non-normal attraction to objects, situations, or individuals) in which a person is sexually attracted to an amputee.

Agalmatophilia: Sexual attraction to mannequins, statues, dolls, or other figured objects.

Anasteemaphilia: Attraction to, or a sexual preference for, a potential partner based on a disproportionate difference in height.

Anililagnia: Attraction by young men (also known as cougar hunters) to older women.

Algolagnia: A perversion (sadism or masochism) exemplified by pleasure and primarily sexual gratification in inflicting or suffering pain.

Altocalciphilia: Being turned on by high heels.

Apotemnophilia: Sexual arousal based on one imagining themselves as an amputee.

Asphyxiophilia: Asphyxiation or strangulation, which is supposed to enhance orgasms.

Autassassinophilia: A paraphilia in which a person is sexually aroused by the thought, or the risk, of being murdered.

Autagonistophilia: Being aroused when on stage or on camera.

Autonepiophilia: Sexual fetish that involves playing the role of an infant in sexual encounters.

Autopedophilia: Sexual fetish that involves playing the role of a child in sexual encounters.

Autoplushophilia: The thought/image of one's self in the form of a plush or anthropomorphized animal (also known as Autozoophilia). These people are also referred to as "plushies" or "furries," and they can't get their jollies unless they are dressed as their favorite stuffed animal.

Autovampirism: Sexual fetish that involves role-playing as a vampire.

Avisodomy: Sex with a bird.

Axillism: Sexually attracted to the smell of a partner's armpit, or using the armpit for sex.

Biastophilia: Sexually assaulting a nonconsenting person, usually a stranger. Also known as raptophilia or, more commonly, rape.

Burusera: A Japanese term for a panty fetish, which is an extremely prevalent fetish in Japan.

Catheterophilia: A sexual perversion that revolves around the insertion of a catheter or other foreign body into the urethra.

Chremastistophilia: Arousal from being charged for sex or sexual role-playing involving robbery.

Chrysophilia: The sexual attraction to gold or gold-colored objects

Choreophilia: The fetish of wanting to dance to achieve orgasm.

Chronophilia: Desire for partners of a widely differing chronological age.

Coprophilia: The paraphilia involving sexual pleasure from excrement.

Coulrophilia: Being aroused by clowns.

Crush fetish: When one becomes sexually aroused while witnessing someone crush objects (i.e. food, small animals, insects) under his or her foot.

Dacryphilia: Sexual arousal from seeing tears or making your partner cry.

Dendrophilia: Attraction to trees.

Ederacinism: Sexual pleasure derived from the thought of tearing out sexual organs by the roots.

Emetophilia: Also known as a puke fetish. Arousal from vomit or vomiting.

Eproctophilia: Also known as a fart fetish. Sexual attraction to human flatulence; mainly straight men attracted to flatulent females.

Erotic asphyxia: A potentially dangerous practice wherein a person heightens sexual enjoyment by cutting off his or her air supply while achieving orgasm. Referred to as auto erotic asphyxiation when done while masturbating.

Erotic lactation: The breastfeeding of an adult, usually a male, by a lactating woman for sexual arousal. Also referred to as Lactaphilia.

Erotophonophilia: Sexual arousal or gratification from the potential death of a human being.

Exhibitionism: Exposing one's genitals to unsuspecting and nonconsenting strangers.

Feederism: Erotic eating, feeding, and weight gain.

Formicophilia: Deriving sexual pleasure from insects crawling on the body, specifically on the genitals.

Forniphilia: Sexual arousal from using your partner as a piece of furniture.

Frotteurism: A paraphilic interest in rubbing, usually one's genitals, against a nonconsenting person or stranger for sexual gratification.

Furverts: People who either sexualize their favorite cartoon characters or dress up in animal costumes and take on the persona of that animal. People who are furverts are commonly called furries.

Gerontophilia: A sexual preference for the elderly.

Gynemimetophilia: The fetish of being sexually aroused by a male role-playing as a female or a transvestite.

Hierophilia: Sexual attraction to religious or sacred objects

Hirsutophilia: A fetish revolving around armpit hair.

Hybristophilia: Often known as the Bonnie and Clyde Syndrome, this is a predatory paraphilia in which sexual arousal, facilitation, and even attainment of orgasm are contingent upon being with a partner known to have committed an aggressive or violent crime.

Inflatophilia: A fetish involving inflatable objects like animals, toys or balloons, and/or deriving sexual pleasure from wearing inflatable suits. These people are often referred to as Looners.

Katoptronophilia: A paraphilia that may include having sex or masturbating in front of mirrors.

Kleptophilia: The state of being sexually aroused by theft; also known as kleptolagnia.

Klismaphilia: Sometimes spelled Klysmaphilia, this refers to the receiving of sexual arousal from enemas.

Liquidophilia: Sexual pleasure from immersing genitals in liquids.

Macrophilia: A paraphilia involving sexual fantasies of being tiny and at the mercy of a giant.

Masochism: A sexual perversion characterized by pleasure in being subjected to pain or humiliation.

Mechanophilia: A paraphilia involving cars or other machines; also called "mechaphilia."

Menophilia: A sexual fascination with menstruation.

Morphophilia: A paraphilia involving attraction to a partner whose bodily characteristics are dramatically different (i.e., giants and dwarves, obese and skinny, etc.).

Mucophilia: Sexual arousal involving mucus.

Mysophilia: A paraphilia involving dirtiness and soiled or decaying things.

Narratophilia: Arousal from talking dirty.

Nasophilia: Getting turned on by someone's nose.

Necrophilia: Also called thanatophilia or necrolagnia, this is the sexual attraction to corpses.

Oculolinctus: The fetish of licking a partner's eyeball. Also referred to as worming.

Odaxelagnia: A paraphilia concerning sexual arousal brought on by biting, or being bitten.

Olfactophilia: Also referred to as Osmolagnia, this is a paraphilia revolving around the smells and odors emanating from the body, especially the genitals.

Omorashi: A Japanese fetish involving sexual attraction to having, or to someone else having, a full bladder.

Paraphilic infantilism: Sexual arousal centered on dressing or being treated like a baby, also known as autonepiophilia or adult baby syndrome.

Partialism: A sexual attraction to specific, but non-genital body parts.

Pecattiphilia: Sexual arousal from performing an act one believes is immoral or a sin.

Pedovestism: Sexual paraphilia obtained by dressing like a child (also autopedophilia).

Peodeiktophilia: Exposing one's penis (also exhibitionism).

Pictophilia: A paraphilia revolving around pornography or erotic art, particularly pictures.

Piquerism: Sexual gratification through stabbing or cutting the body of another person with sharp objects.

Plushophilia: A paraphilia involving stuffed animals. The practitioners are sometimes called plushies, although this term can also refer to a non-sexual affinity to stuffed animals. Also referred to as Ursusagalmatophilia.

Podophilia: Foot fetish.

Ponyplay: A fetish involving human-into-animal transformation.

Psychrophilia: Sexual arousal contingent upon contact with extremely cold objects or watching others freeze.

Pygophilia: The sexualization of the buttocks, especially of the female buttocks. The colloquial term for someone who indulges in this is "ass man."

Pyrophilia: A paraphilia in which the person derives sexual gratification from fire and fire-starting activity. The sexual aspect makes it different from pyromania.

Robotism: A paraphilia based on involving robots in sex play.

Sacofricosis: The process of making a hole in one's pocket to facilitate public masturbation.

Salirophilia: A sexual fetish or paraphilia that involves soiling or disheveling the object of your affection for sexual gratification.

Somnophilia: A paraphilia in which a person sexually gratifies himself with a sleeping partner.

Sthenolagnia: Sexual arousal caused by rubbing, kissing, licking, the muscles of a partner.

Stigmatophilia: A paraphilia involving body piercings and tattoos.

Symphorophilia: A paraphilia in which sexual arousal is contingent upon watching or staging a disaster (e.g. fire, traffic accident, explosions, collapsing buildings).

Tamakeri: Japanese for "ball kicking." This is a sexual fetish in which a female kicks, punches, knees, twists, grabs, or bites a man's testicles.

Telephone scatologia: A fetish involving obscene phone calls.

Teratophilia: A paraphilia devoted to deformed or monstrous people.

Toucherism: Touching an unsuspecting, nonconsenting person with the hand.

Trichophilia: Hair fetishism.

Troilism: Also called cuckoldism, this is a fetish that involves watching one's partner have sex with someone else, sometimes without the third party's knowledge.

Urolagnia: Also called urophilia, undinism, golden showers, and watersports, this is a paraphilia in which sexual excitement is associated with the sight or thought of urine or urination.

Vampirism: A paraphilia in which a person is sexually aroused by blood.

Vorarephilia: Often shortened to "vore," this is a paraphilia where arousal occurs from the idea or fantasy of eating someone, being eaten, or by watching someone eat another person.

Zoophilia: More commonly known as bestiality. People who practice zoophilia are known as zoophiles, zoosexuals, or simply zoos. Zoophilia may also be known as zoosexuality.

Zoosadism: Pleasure (sometimes sexual pleasure) derived from cruelty to animals. The term was coined by Ernest Borneman, who was the president of the German Society for Social-Scientific Sexuality Research from 1982 to 1986.

Zwischenstufe: A German term that refers to a person's attraction to a person of the same sex. This does not necessarily mean that the person is a homosexual or has had sexual relations with a partner of the same sex.

About the Author

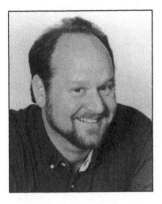 Leland Gregory is the two-time *New York Times* bestselling author of *Stupid American History* and *America's Dumbest Criminals* and is a former writer for Saturday Night Live. Leland has authored nearly thirty books, many of them national bestsellers, including *Stupid History, The Stupid Crook Book*, and *What's The Number for 911?* He has written and sold a screenplay to Disney and optioned another screenplay to Touchstone. He was also co-creator of the nationally syndicated TV series *America's Dumbest Criminals* and recently served as head writer and co-executive producer for the PBS show *The Whole Truth*, which is in negotiations as a series. He's created advertising campaigns for national corporations like Captain D's, International Paper, Cracker Barrel, Dollar General, and AT&T and has contributed to such publications as *Readers Digest, George,* and *Maxim.* He became a nationally recognized political media consultant in 1994 when his work helped a long-shot candidate beat an eighteen-year incumbent. In 2002 he was awarded the prestigious Gold Pollie award for Overall Television Campaigns for his work on a highly publicized Senate race.

Leland is an overall nice guy who has no interesting hobbies.